The Digestive System

R. J. Ryall MB MCh FRCS(Eng)
Consultant Surgeon,
Edgware General Hospital,
Middlesex

With a nursing contribution by
Pat Webb SRN RNT DipSocRes
Senior Nurse, Royal Marsden Hospital
(London and Surrey)

SECOND EDITION

CHURCHILL LIVINGSTONE
EDINBURGH LONDON MELBOURNE AND NEW YORK 1984

CHURCHILL LIVINGSTONE
Medical Division of Longman Group Limited

Distributed in the United States of America by Churchill
Livingstone Inc., 1560 Broadway, New York, N. Y. 10036,
and by associated companies, branches and representatives
throughout the world.

First edition 1973
Second edition 1984

ISBN 0 443 02608 4

British Library Cataloguing in Publication Data
Ryall, R.J.
   The digestive system. — 2nd ed. — (Penguin
   library of nursing)
   1. Digestive organs — Diseases
   2. Gastrointestinal disease nursing
   I. Title
   616.3′0024613   RC802

Library of Congress Cataloging in Publication Data
Ryall, R. J. (Robert James)
   The digestive system.
   (Penguin Library of nursing)
   Bibliography: p.
   Includes index.
   1. Gastrointestinal system — Diseases — Nursing.
   2. Digestive organs — Diseases — Nursing. 3. Gastro-
   intestinal system. I. Webb, Pat (Pat A.) II. Title.
   III. Series. [DNLM: 1. Digestive system — Nurses'
   instruction. 2. Digestive system diseases — Nursing.
   WY 156.5 R988d]
   RC802.R93   1984   616.3   84-3135

Printed in Singapore by Selector Printing Co (Pte) Ltd

To my wife Carmelita

Acknowledgements

We wish to thank the following for permission to use material that has been the basis for some of the illustrations:
For Figures 1, 15, 34, 53, 60, 62, 96, 97: Orbis Publishing Limited, *Mind and Body*. For Figures 2, 66: Churchill Livingstone Ltd, *Illustrated Physiology* by A. B. McNaught and R. Callander. For Figures 11, 43, 66: Churchill Livingstone Ltd, *Textbook of Operative Surgery* by Eric L. Farquharson. For Figures 40, 41, 47, 69, 71, 73: *Nursing Times*. For Figures 18, 79, 80: Key Med Ltd, Specialised Services to Medicine and Industry.

Preface

Gastroenterology today is perhaps one of the most rapidly advancing branches of medical science. If the nurse is to keep abreast of these advances she must have a thorough knowledge of the basic structure and function of the alimentary tract, both in health and disease. An attempt has been made in this book to depart from the traditional textbook presentation of facts, and present instead in narrative style the story of the digestive system.

The level of knowledge is aimed at the student nurse with only a basic understanding of anatomy and physiology. She is encouraged to take a more active part in the care of the patient by having a fuller understanding of the changes which take place when normal function is disturbed.

A nurse's place is on the ward. Her work will be more effective and her job more interesting if she applies her knowledge of anatomy, physiology and pathology to individual patients. In writing these pages, this has been my constant aim. A nurse should be encouraged to seek the reason why.

It is not intended that this book should give a detailed account of all the disease processes which can affect the digestive system. The common conditions that the nurse meets on the ward are presented in the hope that she will be stimulated to further reading. For this reason, further references will be found at the end of the book.

I am grateful to Miss Pat Webb for her invaluable help in the preparation of the second edition of this work. She has included a new chapter on 'Common nursing problems related to disorders of the digestive tract' and has brought up to date the pre- and post-operative nursing care sections of other chapters.

I would like to thank the staff of Churchill Livingstone for their help and constant forbearance during the preparation of this second edition. To Dr Ted Nathan and his colleagues in the Radiological Department of Edgware General Hospital I owe a debt of gratitude for the X-ray illustrations. To my overworked secretary,

Lilian Jenkinson, who has been responsible for much of the manuscript typing, appreciative thanks are due. Lastly, I would like to acknowledge the forbearance of my wife and family, whose constant support enabled me to finish this work.

Middlesex, 1984   R. J. R.

Contents

One
The alimentary tract

The structure of the tract

The function of the alimentary tract is to break down the constituents of food during digestion, to absorb useful substances and reject the surplus.

It is a simple tube measuring approximately nine metres (thirty feet) from end to end. To fit into the human body this tube is either coiled, as is the case in the small intestine, dilated, as in the stomach, or it may occupy a square shape, as in the large intestine.

Different parts of the tube have quite separate roles in the digestion and absorption of food, and are given different names (Figure 1). The first part of the tube is called the *oesophagus*, from the Greek meaning 'to carry food'. It is straight and runs down from the back of the mouth to the entrance of the stomach; it is forty centimetres long. The *stomach* (the dilated part of the tube) is a flask-shaped bag lying transversely in the upper part of the abdominal cavity. It has three distinct sections – some animals have three stomachs. The three parts of the human stomach are the *fundus* or roof of the stomach, the *body* or middle portion and the *antrum*, the cave-like narrow portion leading to the exit which is known as the pylorus (see Figure 35).

The pylorus of the stomach leads into the first part of the small intestine, the *duodenum*, so-called because it is about twelve finger-breadths long. It is shaped like a U lying on its side, and has three parts. The first part is often called the *duodenal cap*, the second part is the *descending portion* and the third part continues as the *jejunum*. The jejunum comprises the first two and a half metres (about eight feet) of the small intestine, whose total length is approximately seven metres (about twenty-two feet). The lower three-fifths of the small intestine, following on from the jejunum, is the *ileum* which runs a winding course through the abdominal cavity (see Figure 67).

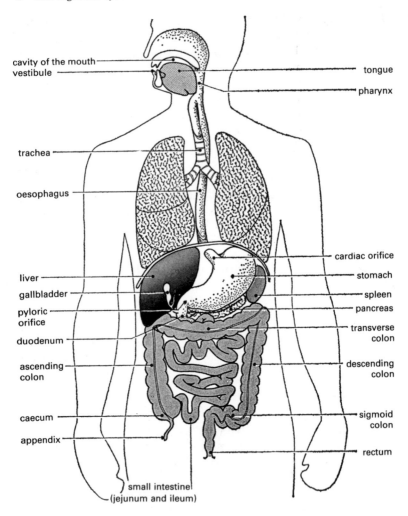

cavity of the mouth
vestibule
tongue
pharynx
trachea
oesophagus
cardiac orifice
liver
stomach
gallbladder
spleen
pyloric orifice
pancreas
duodenum
transverse colon
ascending colon
descending colon
caecum
sigmoid colon
appendix
rectum
small intestine (jejunum and ileum)

Figure 1 The digestive system

The end of the ileum marks the end of the small intestine and the start of the large intestine, which is a much wider tube. The large intestine is also known as the *colon* or large bowel (see Figure 75). The ileum opens into the *caecum*, which is the first part of the colon and literally means a 'blind pouch'. From here, the colon runs up towards the liver and is called the *ascending colon*. The colon then turns through a right angle and continues across the abdominal cavity towards the spleen. Because it runs transversely, it is called the *transverse colon*. At the level of the spleen, it turns through a further right angle and runs down towards the pelvis as the *descending colon*. The portion of the large bowel which lies in the pelvis is called the *pelvic* or *sigmoid colon* (the word 'sigmoid' means S-shaped). Finally, deep down in the pelvis at the level of the middle of the sacrum, the colon straightens out and becomes the *rectum*. The exit from the rectum is through the *anal canal* which is just under four centimetres long. The external orifice, the end of the alimentary tract, is called the *anus*.

The alimentary tract provides fuel to make the other systems of the body work. This fuel is obtained from the food we eat. The tract can be compared to an oil pipeline: at one end very crude oil is pumped in, as the oil flows along the pipe, it is purified and at various stages different fractions of the oil are filtered off. Eventually all the valuable ingredients are taken off, leaving only useless waste products which flow out at the other end.

Muscles of the tract

The alimentary tract is well supplied with muscles in order to propel food along. It also has a mechanism for drawing off the fuel from the food. This filtering mechanism lines the alimentary tract and is called the *mucous membrane* (Figure 2). At different levels in

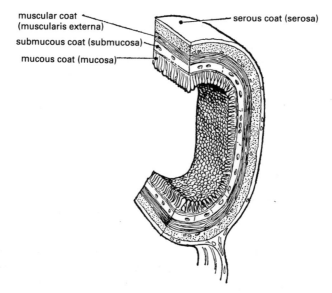

Figure 2 The four layers of the gut wall

the tract, different fractions of the food are filtered off or absorbed, and the mucous membrane differs accordingly. The fuel from the food must eventually reach the blood stream to be transported to the other systems of the body and, for this purpose, the alimentary tract is provided with a rich blood supply.

Once the food is swallowed, the whole digestive process is regulated quite automatically and unconsciously. This regulation is brought about in two ways: firstly, by a system of nerves called *autonomic nerves* and, secondly, by chemical substances called *hormones*.

The arrangement of muscles in the alimentary tract is simple. One layer of muscle encircles the tube and is called the *circular muscle*. When this contracts, the contents of the tube are propelled forwards. This can sometimes be seen in people with a thin abdominal wall as a worm-like movement of the tube, and is known as *peristalsis* (Figure 3). Outside the circular muscle lies a long strip of muscle fibres called the *longitudinal muscle*. When this contracts, the tube gets shorter and fatter, enabling the food to remain in that particular part of the tube for a longer period of time. The stomach has an extra layer of muscle which runs obliquely around its wall. The function of this muscle is to cause a churning movement in the stomach to help break down the food into smaller particles.

At three places in the alimentary tract the circular muscle is very strong and forms ring-like structures called *sphincters* (Figure 4). The word sphincter means 'that which binds tight'. The first is the *pyloric sphincter* at the exit of the stomach. When this contracts, the exit from the stomach is closed so that no food can leave it. When it relaxes, the pylorus opens and the contents of the stomach are propelled onwards to the duodenum.

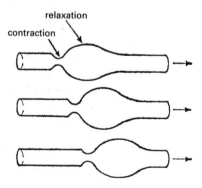

Figure 3 Peristalsis in the small intestine

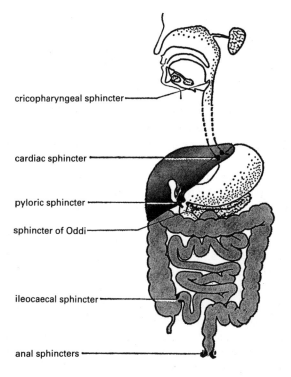

cricopharyngeal sphincter

cardiac sphincter

pyloric sphincter

sphincter of Oddi

ileocaecal sphincter

anal sphincters

Figure 4 The position of the sphincters in the digestive system

The second sphincter or valve is at the junction of the small intestine and colon and is described as the *ileocaecal sphincter*. This sphincter controls the amount of fluid passing into the colon. The third sphincter controls the exit of undigested material at the anus and is therefore called the *anal sphincter*. It is this sphincter which exercises control over bowel movements. It differs from the other two in that it is under voluntary control. If for any reason this sphincter is damaged, then incontinence (involuntary passing of faeces) results. The disease giving rise to this are described in Chapter 9. A further sphincter-like muscle is present at the junction of the oesophagus and the stomach. The main function of this sphincter is to prevent the contents of the stomach from regurgitating into the oesophagus, particularly when the head is lowered.

In the colon the longitudinal muscle is gathered into three bands, each about half a centimetre wide. These bands are shorter than the total length of the colon by about one-sixth, giving it a slightly puckered appearance.

Mucous membrane

The mucous membrane is perhaps the most important structure in the alimentary tract – it is the active filter which transfers the essential chemicals from the alimentary tract to the blood stream. The mucous membrane is not only a lining – it also contains glands which pour substances into the tube to help in the digestion of food. When the food is digested, it is broken down into minute particles, and the mucous membrane transfers these particles into the narrow extensions of blood vessels called *capillaries*. Digestion is a continuous process, so the mucous membrane has a different structure in different parts of the tract.

In the oesophagus, where food simply passes through, the mucous membrane is strong and tough and is the strongest layer of the oesophagus as it must withstand a great deal of wear and tear. When viewed under a microscope it is seen to be made up of several layers of cells called *squamous* cells. These are not unlike the cells of the skin.

The lining of the stomach is more specialized because it must produce acid, mucus, pepsin and a hormone called gastrin to help digestion. This lining is known as the *gastric epithelium* and performs different functions in the three parts of the stomach. The epithelium in the fundus produces mucus, the epithelium in the body is responsible for acid production, whilst that in the antrum produces the hormone gastrin. These will be discussed later in relation to the functions or physiology of the stomach (see p. 59).

The lining of the small intestine is rather beautiful. If it is viewed under the microscope, it can be seen to be folded into millions of tiny finger-like processes called *villi*. These wave to and fro when fluid passes over them. They are hollow and contain a capillary and another tiny vessel called a *lacteal*. The lining of the colon is the same as that of the rectum. Its chief properties are those of water absorption and mucus production.

Blood supply

The whole of the alimentary tract has a very rich blood supply which carries away the products of digestion. It is so important that, if the blood vessels supplying any part are damaged or blocked near the tube, the neighbouring blood vessels will take over their duties. However, if a major blood vessel is blocked before it divides

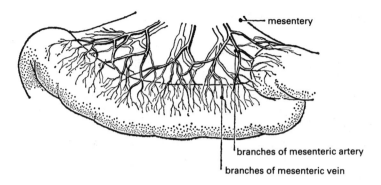

Figure 5 The terminal blood supply of the small intestine

into its branches, the blood supply may be cut off and part of the intestine may die. This may occur especially in elderly people.

The arterial supply to the alimentary tract is in the form of several large arteries arising from the *aorta* (the body's main artery). The main artery to the stomach arises from the aorta just below the diaphragm and is called the *coeliac artery*. From this main source, branches go out to all parts of the stomach. The arterial supply to the small intestine comes from a branch of the aorta called the *superior mesenteric artery*. The small intestine is suspended from the back of the abdominal wall by a membranous fold called the *mesentery* and the artery runs along this, which explains its name (Figure 5). This artery also supplies the right and transverse colon by branches called *colic branches*. Thus, if the superior mesenteric artery becomes blocked at its origin, a large part of the alimentary tract loses its blood supply. The left sides of the colon and rectum obtain their blood from a large artery called the *inferior mesenteric artery*.

These three arteries divide and subdivide and join with each other in the mesentery to form arcades, and this is the 'safety device' which ensures a continuous supply. When the arteries approach the bowel wall, they penetrate the muscle layers, getting smaller and smaller until eventually they reach the mucous membrane in the form of very narrow capillaries. The enormous network of capillaries in the alimentary tract is so large that it is given the special name *splanchnic bed*. If all the capillaries were opened up at the same time all the blood in the human body could be contained in this 'bed'.

The capillaries in the mucous membrane unite to form tiny veins. It is in these veins that the products of digestion are transported

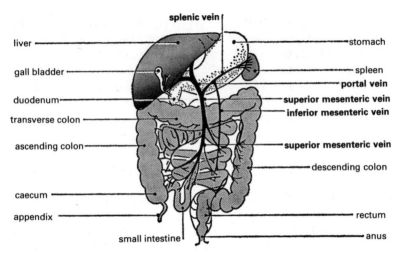

Figure 6 The veins of the digestive system

away from the alimentary canal to the sites where they are used. The ultimate destination is the liver, which is the main chemical factory and storehouse of the body. The veins get larger as they travel away from the alimentary tract in the mesentery and they all eventually join to form the *portal vein* (Figure 6) which drains into the liver and which is part of the total *portal system* of veins linking the alimentary tract with the other internal organs.

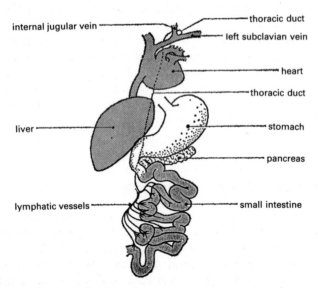

Figure 7 The lymphatics from the gut

A further system of vessels runs alongside the arteries and veins in the mesentery. These are the *lymph vessels* and are the main route by which fat is carried away from the alimentary tract (Figure 7). The lymph vessels pass through a series of filters called *lymph glands* and eventually join the main lymph vessel called the *thoracic duct*. This travels up through the back of the chest and empties itself into a large vein at the root of the left side of the neck.

Control by the nervous system

The automatic self-regulation of digestion is brought about through a vast system of automatic nerves, called the sympathetic and parasympathetic nerves. These originate in the brain and travel down to the alimentary tract through a system of relays or knots of nerve cells called *ganglia*. The nerves finally reach every part of the alimentary tract via the mesentery. In general, the sympathetic nerves control the amount of blood flowing through the intestine at any one time. After a meal, for example, more blood will be needed, so the sympathetic nerves cause the vessels to dilate. Conversely, during strenuous exercises the muscles will have priority so that the large splanchnic bed will be closed down. The parasympathetic system, in general, controls the movement of food through the alimentary tract by contracting and relaxing the muscles of the tube during peristalsis, and by opening and closing the sphincters at appropriate times.

The nervous system also governs the secretion of acid in the stomach, through the mediation of the vagus nerve, which is part of the autonomic nervous system. During periods of stress or anxiety, more impulses are sent down the vagus nerve, so more acid is produced. This is commonly experienced as 'butterflies in the stomach', but is also important in relation to peptic ulcers (see p. 69).

The process of digestion

Fuel is obtained from the food we eat. The three basic kinds of food are proteins, carbohydrates and fats. These, when taken by mouth, consist of very complex chemical substances. Before they are transported into the blood stream they must be broken down into simpler chemical substances and dissolved. This is the essence of the process of digestion.

Digestion starts in the mouth. *Saliva*, the fluid produced by salivary glands, aids mastication. It also contains an enzyme (a substance which speeds up or slows down a chemical reaction) called *ptyalin* which helps to break down starch (a carbohydrate) into smaller carbohydrate fractions. Then the food passes through the oesophagus, where nothing important happens to it, and on to the stomach. But the sight and smell of food has already stimulated the gastric mucosa of the stomach to secrete the gastric juice. This juice contains:

(a) a strong acid called *hydrochloric acid*;

(b) an enzyme, called *pepsin*, which breaks down proteins;

(c) a sticky substance, called *mucin*, which helps to dissolve chemicals and neutralize excess acid.

When the food enters the stomach, it is thoroughly mixed and dissolved. The presence of food stimulates the antrum to produce a hormone called *gastrin*, and this helps to produce more gastric juice. Eventually all the food is dissolved, producing a fluid called *acid chyme*, which has the consistency of very thin porridge. When this stage is reached, the pyloric sphincter opens and the fluid is squirted into the duodenum.

Bile, produced by the liver and stored in the gall bladder, also enters the duodenum, through a small opening in the second part. Through the same opening pours the secretion of the *pancreas*, an important gland lying behind the stomach and producing three very valuable enzymes:

(a) *trypsin*, which breaks down proteins still further;

(b) *amylase*, which breaks down starch still further;

(c) *lipase*, which converts fat into its constituents chemical parts.

The duodenal juice therefore contains a mixture of bile and pancreatic juice and is alkaline, in contrast to the gastric juice which is acidic. The pouring of pancreatic juice into the duodenum is stimulated by another hormone (*secretin*) secreted by the duodenal mucosa. The bile digests fat by reducing it to a fine emulsion.

The food, at this stage, is almost completely digested, and now passes into the small intestine, where it comes into contact with the intestinal juice called *succus entericus*. This contains more important enzymes which complete the process of digestion. In the small intestine the complex proteins have now been broken down into amino acids, the carbohydrates into the simple sugars glucose and fructose, and the fats into tiny particles of glycerol and fatty acids called *chylomicrons*. They are now all absorbed or transported into the blood stream through the villi of the small intestine, and this explains why the villi and tiny blood vessels are so closely related. Almost complete absorption of the products of digestion and of other materials such as water, salts, vitamins and minerals occurs in the small intestine. Reduced absorption of foodstuffs from the small intesine may be due to insufficient intake, inadequate digestion from lack of pancreatic or other juices, lack of materials such as bile salts to promote absorption, an abnormal state of the wall of the small intestine, or an insufficient length of the small intestine – as may occur if some of it has been removed surgically.

It takes three and a half hours for the food to travel from the mouth to the ileocaecal valve. The main function of this valve is to prevent the fluid contents of the ileum from passing too rapidly into the caecum, and the contents of the tract are held up at this point for about an hour. However, an important substance, vitamin B_{12}, is absorbed at this site. When the valve opens, the fluid chyme passes into the caecum. Most of the important chemicals have now been extracted from the food, so the contents of the caecum and ascending colon are merely the residue. But, if this residue were passed out in its fluid form, the body would very quickly become dehydrated. One of the functions of the colon therefore is to absorb water from this residue and return it to the blood stream, from which much of it first originated as various secretions higher up in the alimentary tract. Most of the absorption of water occurs in the caecum and ascending colon, and very little in the transverse and descending colon. The other important function of the colon is to secrete *mucus*, which facilitates the passage of faeces. This mucus also passes on the unabsorbed fractions of ingested iron, calcium, phosphate, etc. When the contents of the colon reach the sigmoid colon, about eighteen hours after the food was eaten, further absorption of water occurs, and this gives the faeces (the residue left after the absorption of food and the intestinal secretions) their normal consistency. Some foods, especially if they contain cellulose, a very indigestible substance, pass out unchanged in the faeces. Faeces are evacuated in the act of *defaecation*.

A considerable volume of fluid is necessary for digestion. This fluid, made up of gastric juice, bile, pancreatic juice and small-intestinal fluid, comes mainly from the blood and passes, via the digestive glands, into the lumen of the bowel. It is finally returned to the blood from both the small intestine and the colon. This exchange of water is called *internal fluid turnover* and, on average, amounts to as much as eight or nine litres a day in the alimentary tract. In addition, water is constantly being formed in all tissues as an end-product of the burning or oxidation of foodstuffs by the cells. This amounts to approximately 300 ml per day. Food itself, depending on the diet, contains about 1000 ml of water per day. Water lost in the faeces amounts to about 100 ml daily in the normal person. This loss is increased in diarrhoea. Thus the alimentary tract plays a significant part in the maintenance of the body's internal environment (the *milieu interieur*).

The peritoneum

The abdomen is lined with tissue called the *peritoneum*, which is a strong, colourless, serous membrane. At various places it is folded over the *viscera* (the internal organs), forming a complete covering for the stomach, liver, spleen, small intestine, transverse colon, pelvic colon and upper part of the rectum (see Figure 47). It also partially covers the ascending and descending colon. The peritoneum holds the viscera in position by its folds, some of which form the mesenteries, which have already been mentioned. Other folds, called the *omenta*, are attached to the stomach. That part of the peritoneum lining the abdominal wall is called the *parietal peritoneum*. The space between the parietal and visceral peritoneum is called the *peritoneal cavity*; this has two important compartments called the *greater* and *lesser sacs*.

In general, the alimentary tract is insensitive to touch or cutting but, if it is stretched or pulled, pain, known as *visceral pain* is experienced. This is not localized in any one place, and patients usually have difficulty in describing its character. The peritoneum lining the abdominal wall (the parietal peritoneum) is largely supplied with nerves which are as sensitive as the nerves on our skin so, if it is stimulated excessively, a sharp and well-localized pain (*somatic pain*) is experienced. These differences are important in various diseases of the alimentary tract, to be discussed later.

Development of the alimentary tract

In the foetus the alimentary tract is formed as a straight tube, developed from the middle (mesodermal) layer of cells in the embryo. This tube becomes divided into three parts called the foregut, midgut and hindgut, which are suspended from the main artery (aorta). Each part has its own artery. The artery to the foregut becomes the coeliac artery, that to the midgut the superior mesenteric artery, and that to the hindgut the inferior mesenteric artery. As the tube gets longer, the midgut becomes extruded outside the foetus for part of its development. Nourishment for the development of the tract is obtained from the yolk sac through a duct called the *vitello-intestinal duct*. Sometimes part of this duct remains in adult life, arising from the lower part of the ileum, and is called *Meckel's diverticulum*. Later in development, the midgut returns to the peritoneal cavity of the foetus and is rotated and twisted to accommodate itself. This explains the position of the alimentary tract in the peritoneal cavity.

Developing from the foregut, the stomach and first part of the duodenum retain their blood supply from the coeliac artery. The remainder of the duodenum, small intestine, caecum, ascending colon and the right half of the transverse colon develop from the midgut, and all these structures are supplied by the original artery, the superior mesenteric artery. The left side of the transverse colon, the descending colon, the sigmoid colon and the rectum develop from the hindgut and they all receive their blood from the inferior mesenteric artery. These three arteries arise from the front of the aorta.

Two

Common nursing problems related to disorders of the digestive tract

The digestive tract is a dynamic system involved in processing the food we eat to provide resources, particularly energy and nutrients, required by every living cell. It also plays a vital role in the control of fluid balance in the body.

Eating and drinking, and the passage of waste resulting from digestion and metabolism, are fundamental functions of our normal lives. Eating and drinking is also an enjoyable social habit for the majority. When we think about food, and the pleasure of eating, or when we see or smell food as it is being prepared, the nervous system registers the fact and stimulates releasing factors which prepare our digestive tract to receive and break down the food by the use of its many gastric juices and enzymes.

When we are well, much of our day is structured around mealtimes. These have two functions: of providing a regular intake of food and of satisfying social needs.

Nursing history and assessment

In addition to the collection of data relating to physical factors the nursing history should include the usual eating and drinking habits and preferences of the patient. Foods which may disturb normal function should be noted, as these may have significance both for the patient's present physical condition and for dietary consideration whilst he is in hospital.

If pain is expressed as a symptom, it needs to be assessed in respect of exact site, frequency and duration. Pain is a subjective experience, and it is, therefore, very difficult to accurately represent. An effective way of exactly locating pain is to ask the patient to mark the areas where pain is felt on a body outline diagram (Figure 8). Descriptive terms can then be used to specify the

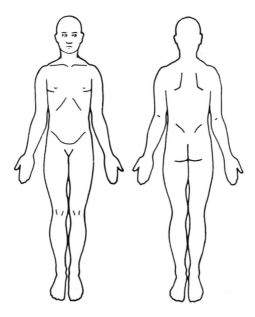

Figure 8

particular sensation: for example, burning, cutting, cramp-like or ache.

Pain may not be the only sensation that requires a base-line evaluation in assessing the patient. 'Indigestion' is a descriptive term that may also be ambiguous, meaning something quite different to the patient and the nurse. 'A burning pain in my chest before I eat' is a much more useful description and gives a great deal more information.

Details of bowel movements and the appearance of faeces may be very important in some cases, and are significant in all patients with disorders of the gastro-intestinal tract. Failure to communicate precise details is a common problem.

Frequent bowel movements, for some people, may mean that stools are passed three times in twenty-four hours if it is normal to have bowel movements only every other day. Diarrhoea and frequent bowel movements are often considered to be the same thing by patients and by some nurses. Normal stools passed more frequently than usual may be described as persistent diarrhoea when clearly this may not be the case. The nurse should obtain and record an accurate description of exactly what is happening.

Further assessment should be made by the nurse of the condition of the patient's skin and mouth. Dehydration and poor nourishment can often be identified in this way. Such observations are vital base-lines for planning and providing care in the future.

The team approach to care

An assessment will also be made by the doctor. The same questions need not necessarily be asked twice but information should be available for the nursing assessment from a nursing history to ensure that competent care is negotiated and delivered.

The nurse may ask other questions when recording the patient's history, all of which are relevant to the total picture she will build up of this individual within his normal home environment. This will help her deduce how his personality and life-style may have contributed to his current illness. From the nursing history, current needs or problems can be identified and potential problems planned for. The nurse, patient and close relatives plan together, allowing the patient to feel in control of his situation from the outset and to be actively involved in regaining health throughout his illness.

The serving and presentation of meals is very important for patients when they are in hospital. In the strange environment and social disorder in which they find themselves, some normality may be retained by the routine of mealtimes. If the ward is one where some patients may be disturbed even by the smell of food, provision should be made to temporarily segregate those eating normally from those unable to do so. The sensory input of sight and smell of food is powerful, and although this is usually a very positive function it can be a very unpleasant one if other patients are nauseated by it. If appetite is poor and needs to be encouraged, small, attractive servings of food are best. Sensitivity to the patient's individual needs is very important. Mealtimes do give some shape to the hospital day, and restore some normality to an otherwise strange existence.

Investigation prior to diagnosis

If the patient is hospitalised for investigation and treatment the nurse should be sensitive to the anxieties and discomfort caused by some of the investigations. They may not be painful, but they disrupt a patient's life and will cause apprehension. An everyday event for the nurse can be a major milestone for the patient.

The period between the first out-patient appointment and the eventual confirmatory diagnosis may be agonising for the patient and relatives. Fear of the unknown causes extreme rises in anxiety levels, and opportunity for information exchange between the patient and those caring for him must be frequent to allow any anxieties to be aired and questions to be asked. During the period of investigation the hospital patient will spend much time waiting for results. If investigation is completed prior to hospitalisation, the patient is able to go home to normal living and the family circle in the evenings. Such support will help him to talk though his fears and worries in familiar surroundings. But for the inpatient the nurse must be a listener and information provider during this difficult time. Information-giving paced by the patient himself is ideal. At times, the nurse may feel unable to give accurate information due to lack of knowledge. She may have to find out or ask someone else to provide the details. The nurse should be honest with the patient and tell him she cannot answer his questions. But under no circumstances should she leave the patient who is asking for help without referring him to another member of staff who can help, as this may be the only time that he has the courage to ask. If communication channels are not kept open, the patient may be worrying unnecessarily, and this will not help him to prepare himself for his future treatment. If a patient appears to be withdrawn and is not asking for any information about himself, however basic, the nurse may have to make the opportunity for him to talk, by initiating conversations which will give him the 'licence' to ask questions.

The waiting time

Specific investigations are mentioned in later chapters, as they relate to specific organs. Adequate preparation for these is most important. Failure to do what is required will only cause subsequent delays for the patient. The nurse, by taking short cuts in her preparation, will ultimately be doing the patient a disservice. Sensitivity to individual patients is important even in the preparation for investigation. For example, bowel preparation may cause little disruption to one individual, but cause extreme anxiety and discomfort to another. No two patients are alike, and each needs to be assessed and treated individually with patience and understanding.

When there is no new information or treatment to offer until results are known, it is easy to ignore the waiting patient and spend more time with those who are actively requiring the nurse's skills. However, the nurse should allow time to spend with this waiting patient. Her listening and encouragement are just as important to him as management of intravenous fluids and monitoring of vital signs may be to the new post-operative patient. The nurse will learn gradually how to manage her time to accommodate the needs of all the patients in her care during each of her periods of work.

The plan for treatment

When diagnosis is confirmed, the treatment plan will be established in consultation with the patient. The nurse may be called upon to constantly reinforce this information, and she should make herself familiar with all the details so that she can feel confident to do so.

Common problems found in patients with disorders of the gastro-intestinal tract are outlined below: details should be obtained from physiology textbooks.

1. Fluid balance

The body needs fluid in order to function; it preserves just enough fluid for its needs, discarding any excesses. This is done by a complex system of functions in many different organs, each playing a vital role in maintaining the internal environment of the body. The gastro-intestinal tract is particularly important in this respect. Secretions into the gastro-intestinal tract, from the salivary glands through into the intestines, amount to over 8 litres in every 24 hours. The digestive juices are secreted in response to stimuli, either before food is ingested, or after, or both before and after, and are responsible for the chemical breakdown of food in the process of digestion to metabolism.

Most of these juices are reabsorbed for use again, but where there has been surgery to the tract, fluid may escape from a fistula, an ileostomy, or a temporary drainage tube. If this fluid is not replaced by intravenous therapy, or if appropriate, nasogastric feeding, the patient will become severely dehydrated.

Depending on where the fluid escapes from, there may also be severe electrolyte loss (acid or alkali loss as the pH changes along the course of the tract) and subsequent electrolyte imbalance with dehydration. Metabolic acidosis or alkalosis may occur and be life-threatening if it is not corrected.

The nurse must meticulously measure and report all drainage from any body cavity, drainage tube, or wound, and may in some circumstances be asked to test the fluid for its acidity or alkalinity with a suitable reagent.

Fluid intake should also be measured and monitored accurately. If intravenous therapy is being administered, the prescribed regimes should be strictly adhered to and the underlying principle of treatment understood. Sometimes it may be necessary not only to measure all fluids accurately, but also to weigh the patient at the same time each day and in the same condition (if weighing just the patient, he should be dressed in the same clothes each time; if weighing the bed, this must be in the same condition on each occasion).

Weight and fluid measurements together give as accurate a picture as possible of fluid loss and gain. 1 litre of fluid weighs approximately one kilogram, so an unplanned weight loss or gain of this amount would indicate severe disturbance in normal function.

It is absolutely essential that fluid balance is taken seriously. Failure to do so is negligence and may cause severe harm to the patient.

2. Nutrition

Insufficient emphasis is placed upon the nutritional needs of the patient both before and after surgery. There is ample evidence to show that a balanced diet with adequate levels of all basic foods puts the patient in the best position to regain health during and following treatment, particularly surgery. The patient will be malnourished if nausea and vomiting has been a problem for some time, or if the patient is on a low income, or is elderly or disabled in any way and therefore unable to care for himself adequately. If this is the case, total parenteral nutrition may be established prior to major surgery. This is a way of giving highly concentrated solution intravenously to maintain the nutritional needs of an individual over a period of time (refer to other texts for detail).

If the patient is malnourished, healing following surgery will be affected and restoration to normal health and mobilisation will be delayed. The nurse can significantly contribute to restoring and maintaining adequate nutrition if she understands how vital this is.

Whatever method of nutrition is decided for the patient, ensuring that he receives this is as important a part of his total care as recording his blood-pressure or measuring his fluid intake and output.

3. Body image

Everyone has an image of his or her body. The surgical patient who has undergone an operation for the removal or remodelling of organs has to cope with the additional trauma of an altered body image.

A change in hairstyle or the eruption of spots is a common disturbance of this image that most people have experienced. But if this mental image is drastically disturbed it may take a very long time to restore equilibrium.

Surgical wounds cause scars. It may take patients some time to accept the presence of these blemishes. But when a limb or breast is removed the patient's appearance to the world and to herself is profoundly altered.

In digestive tract disorders, the most significant change to a patient's appearance is when an ileostomy or colostomy is raised onto the abdominal surface. It may take many months or years for the patient to accept this new image. Some never do accept it, and full health in this respect is not restored. A compromise may be reached, and the stoma may be recognised by the patient as a disability. Much of the nurse's time must, therefore, be devoted to this aspect of her total patient care.

This chapter is only an introduction to some of the matters of nursing management of patients with disorders of the digestive tract. Its aim is to stimulate thought and encourage the reader to search other texts in more depth to arrive at a full understanding of the implications of nursing these patients and of giving excellent care.

Three
The mouth and salivary glands

The tongue and saliva

The tongue (Figure 9) can provide a great deal of information about the general state of the alimentary tract. This is why the doctor usually inspects the patient's tongue. A healthy tongue is pink and moist. This moistness is preserved by the *saliva*, which bathes the inside of the mouth. Saliva is secreted by the *salivary glands* (Figure 10), which are situated in the cheeks and pour their secretions into the mouth via well-defined channels or *ducts*. The openings of these ducts can be seen by looking carefully inside the mouth. The largest gland, the *parotid*, opens into the mouth on the upper cheek opposite the second molar tooth on either side. Underneath the tongue, the openings of the *submandibular salivary glands* can be seen situated close together on either side of the fraenum of the tongue. Also opening into the floor of the mouth are many ducts from the *sublingual salivary glands*, which lie beneath it. The salivary juice is clear and watery and prevents the infection which would occur if the mouth became too dry. Many stimuli result in the secretion of saliva, but the most powerful of them is the sight (or taste) of food.

In addition to keeping the mouth moist, the salivary juice has other important uses. It contains the enzyme ptyalin, which starts the process of digestion of starch while food is chewed. (Other enzymes in saliva help to destroy bacteria.) Saliva also moistens the food so that it is swallowed more easily.

The appearance of the tongue provides valuable indications of the state of the digestive system, and the nurse should look at every patient's tongue and note any abnormalities. The observations should be recorded. If this is done as part of the nursing assessment, when admitting a patient, it will provide a base-line for future comparisons. It is most important, therefore, that reporting is clear and comprehensive and concise. For example: . . . . 'tongue

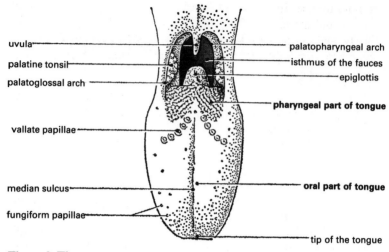

Figure 9 The tongue

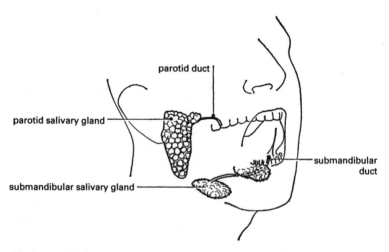

Figure 10 The salivary glands

dry and furry; teeth needing dental assessment; obvious lack of saliva, and some small ulcerated lesions on the inner aspect of the top lip'. Such a record gives a great deal of useful information which can be used to plan mouth-care and as a base-line for monitoring progress. Among the changes which may take place are:

(a) *A dry tongue*; the most common cause is probably persistent breathing through the mouth. However, any disease which causes an excessive loss of water from the body (dehydration) will result in a dry tongue. In this way the body conserves water for more vital organs, and the salivary glands do not secrete. The patient will feel thirsty and, if he can drink, all is well. But sometimes this is forbidden for medical or surgical reasons. Oral hygiene is thus extremely important in an ill patient.

(b) *A brown furred tongue*; this generally means that the body is accumulating the waste products of digestion rather than excreting them. Common examples are prolonged constipation and a condition called *uraemia*, which results from failure of the kidneys to excrete the end-product of the digestion of proteins.

(c) *A smooth glazed tongue*; the tongue, like every other organ in the body, has an outer skin or *epithelium*; if this epithelium is to remain healthy, the body must receive an adequate amount of vitamins daily. This is normally ensured by a correct diet. If, however, the diet lacks vitamins A, B and C, the epithelium will become very thin and the tongue will appear very smooth. Certain *anaemias*, in which the blood becomes low in certain minerals, will cause similar changes by depriving the tongue of nourishment.

Diseases of the tongue

Inflammation of the tongue is known as *glossitis* and may be acute or chronic.

Acute glossitis

This is not a very common condition, but it can be quite serious. The cardinal signs of inflammation are pain, swelling, heat and redness. A swollen tongue may fill the mouth and the throat, blocking the airway and causing death from suffocation. A sting from a wasp may have this result. Other causes of acute glossitis are infection of the tongue, particularly by bacteria known as strep-tococci, certain forms of anaemia and blood diseases, particularly the leukaemias. A sore tongue may be an undesirable side-effect of drugs commonly used in hospitals, a common example being ascorbic acid tablets. Others are the various drugs used in the treatment of malignant disease.

Treatment

This depends on the cause. For example, a patient whose tongue has been stung by a wasp should have ice packs applied to his tongue to reduce the swelling. An antihistamine drug will help to neutralize the poison from the wasp-sting. However, the most important complication that can arise is asphyxia, so the necessary preparations should always be made in case an urgent *tracheostomy* (an artificial opening into the windpipe) should be necessary. If the patient shows signs of respiratory distress, the tongue should be hooked forwards, thereby opening up the space behind the tongue (the *nasopharynx*).

Chronic glossitis

The most common cause of chronic glossitis is syphilis. At first the tongue is red, firm and fissured, but later it becomes white and cracked. This condition is called *leukoplakia*. The importance of leukoplakia is that it is a pre-cancerous condition – if it is left untreated, a cancer may develop in one of the cracks or fissures. Leukoplakia can also occur in any part of the mouth as a result of chronic irritation from jagged teeth, septic tooth roots or ill-fitting dentures.

Treatment

As the most important complication of chronic glossitis and of leukoplakia is the development of cancer, the affected area will always be excised and sent to the laboratory so that the tissue can be examined under the microscope. If the patient is suffering from syphilis this will also be treated. If broken or jagged teeth are the cause, they will be removed. After any operation of the tongue, feeding may be a problem. This is discussed in more detail on page 29.

Tumours of the tongue

There are two basic types of tumour, *benign* and *malignant*.

Benign tumours

The benign tumours are harmless but, if they occur on the tongue, they may cause discomfort during mastication of food. The patient has an irritable nodule on his tongue and so will seek medical advice. The two common benign tumours are:

(a) *Papilloma*: this is a simple overgrowth of the outer lining or epithelium of the tongue and commonly occurs on the tip.

(b) *Angioma*: this is a simple tumour whose cells tend to form blood vessels, so bleeding is a common symptom of this form of tumour. If the angioma is situated on the edge of the tongue, it may be trapped between the teeth and cause a slight haemorrhage.

These tumours may be cured by simple excision. The tongue is richly supplied with blood vessels and nerves and therefore bleeds very freely when cut. Minor operations on the tongue are best carried out under a general anaesthetic. In this way all bleeding can be stopped before the patient is returned to the ward. Because it has such a rich blood supply, the tongue heals very rapidly and the patient need only stay in hospital for 24 hours. In the post-operative period, the nurse should ensure that a clear airway is maintained and that bleeding does not recommence.

Malignant tumours

This is a serious condition and usually comes to the doctor's notice as a painful ulcer. Syphilis and leukoplakia are predisposing factors, but any source of chronic irritation of the tongue, if left untreated for a long time, may lead to the development of a carcinoma. In the past, hot smoke from clay pipes, and irritation of the edge of the tongue from broken septic teeth were common causes, but both of these causes have largely been eradicated and the incidence of carcinoma of the tongue has been reduced. The diagnosis is easily made. Usually by the time the patient seeks medical advice ulceration has occurred and he will complain of pain. However, the pain may be referred to the ear, rather than occurring in the tongue. Malignant ulcers are easily identified because they have a characteristic base and edge. The base of the ulcer feels hard and is usually covered with a foul-smelling slough. The edge is turned over (everted). Other non-malignant ulcers, such as dental and tuberculous ulcers, have different appearances. But the diagnosis is not made on appearance alone. A small sample of cells (a *biopsy*) is taken from the growing edge, and the diagnosis is confirmed under the microscope. If the carcinoma is advanced, the patient may not be able to protrude his tongue. As a result of the irritation of the growth, salivation may be excessive and the patient may dribble. Secondary infection is also usually present.

If left untreated, the carcinoma will spread. All carcinomas spread by three different routes. As the tumour grows, it will first

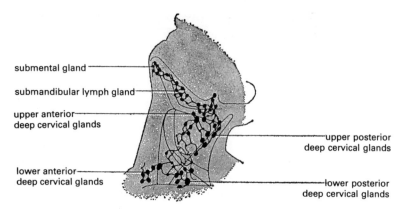

submental gland

submandibular lymph gland

upper anterior
deep cervical glands

upper posterior
deep cervical glands

lower anterior
deep cervical glands

lower posterior
deep cervical glands

Figure 11 Lymphatic drainage of the neck

extend directly into the neighbouring tissues. Secondly, tumour cells can migrate into the lymph vessels draining the organ (Figure 11) and from there to the adjacent lymph nodes where the cells are trapped, consequently enlarging the lymph nodes. Thirdly, if the tumour ulcerates into a blood vessel, cancer cells can be carried in the blood to distant parts of the body and give rise to secondary cancer deposits. A carcinoma of the tongue can extend into the tissues of the neck giving rise to a hard fixed mass. The tongue drains its lymph to nodes which are situated on either side of the neck, and these may therefore enlarge and harden.

If left untreated, the patient with carcinoma of the tongue will invariably die. As a result of the pain and the increase of size of the tumour in the mouth, swallowing will become impossible, and starvation and exhaustion will result. Inhaling septic material from the mouth may cause bronchopneumonia and lead to death. Sometimes, the patient may suffer a massive fatal secondary haemorrhage from the growth.

Treatment

Since prevention is better than cure, vital preventive measures are good oral hygiene and dental care. In addition, two methods of treatment, surgery and radiotherapy, are available for dealing with established cases. Growths in the anterior two-thirds of the tongue can be treated by either method, whilst growths in the posterior third are usually treated by radiotherapy.

Before any surgery is undertaken, it is absolutely essential that the mouth should be as clean as possible. All septic teeth must be removed, even if this means extracting all the teeth. The patient must be taught oral hygiene, and the nurse should ensure that frequent mouth washes of hydrogen peroxide or glycerine of thymol are given.

Each patient should be encouraged to carry out as much of his own mouth care as he is capable of. If he is able to wash his own mouth frequently, then there may be no need for the nurse to clean his mouth for him. Similarly, if a more thorough oral toilet is required there is no reason why the patient should not do this for himself provided he is adequately instructed and supervised. Having your mouth cleaned by someone else is an unpleasant sensation, and should be avoided if possible. However, when it is required, the comfort and refreshment it gives and the help in preventing oral infections are well worth the effort on the part of the nurse and the temporary unpleasant sensation for the patient. Sometimes it is necessary to carry out regular, systematic cleansing of the mouth. If the patient has dentures these must regularly be removed and thoroughly cleansed. The major complications following surgery are infection and secondary haemorrhage, so a surgeon would not operate on an infected mouth.

Excision or removal of the tongue is a very mutilating operation and it is rarely performed, as radiotherapy gives equally good results. If, however, the lymph nodes in the neck are affected, these are usually removed surgically as radiotherapy to the lymph nodes has given disappointing results. This operation is carried out after the treatment to the primary tumour in the tongue has been completed. All the nodes from the base of the skull on the affected side to the collar bone (the *clavicle*) are removed 'en bloc'. This is called a 'block dissection' of the neck (Figure 12).

Radiotherapy is always the doctor's first choice of treatment for carcinoma of the tongue. The same care regarding cleanliness of the mouth should be taken when radiotherapy is used as when surgery

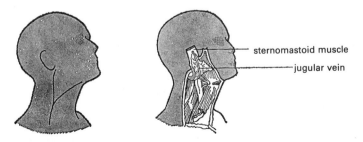

Figure 12 Block dissection of the lymph glands in the neck

is involved. In the anterior two-thirds of the tongue *radium needles* are implanted into the tumour. The most serious complications that can result during treatment with radium needles is loss of one of the needles and, for this reason, each needle has a thread attached to it. These threads are securely attached to the face and one of the nurse's most important duties is to inspect and count the threads regularly to check that a radium needle has not been swallowed. When the needles are removed, the reaction to the radium may be quite severe and the nurse should constantly watch for the occurrence of secondary haemorrhage or bleeding.

When bleeding occurs, attempts should be made by the nurse to arrest it immediately. Holding the tongue firmly with a gauze swab and exerting pressure with the fingers is the best action to take. This is not as easy as it sounds, either for the nurse to do, or for the patient to tolerate, and it is only a temporary measure. However, the prime aim is to prevent inhalation of blood, and subsequent compromising of the airway. The nurse should support the patient in an upright position, with head tilted forwards or, if shocked, in the left lateral position, so that any bleeding can drain easily into a vomit bowl. She should send for help, but must stay with the patient and try to comfort and calm him in this frightening situation. If bleeding is severe and persisting the bleeding points may have to be sealed, by using diathermy or some similar technique, under general anaesthesia.

In growths of the posterior third of the tongue radiotherapy is given as tele-radiation. A cobalt unit emits a beam of radiation and directs it on to the growth.

Pre-operative nursing care

Every patient who has to undergo an operation on his mouth, especially if it involves the tongue, will be particularly concerned about whether his speech will be affected, whether he will be able to swallow and how painful the post-operative period will be. The nurse should explain in simple terms what to expect. Reassurance at this time will instil a confidence that will make the post-operative nursing, more manageable. This is all part of a nurse's role – to provide information for her patients. Preparing a patient for the sequence of events to come helps to allay anxiety and makes the patient feel more in control of the situation. Information is best given verbally and then followed up by something in writing. Written information may be handwritten by the nurse or a printed leaflet specially prepared for the situation. Drawing simple diagrams, or showing pictures of equipment to be used, will allay rather than increase anxiety. Fear of the unknown is much greater than fear of the known.

Post-operative nursing care

In the immediate post-operative period, the maintenance of a clear airway is the first essential. Noisy respiration (*stridor*) in this period is the first clue that the airway may be blocked and the most common reason for this is that the tongue has fallen back, blocking the throat (Figure 13). If this happens, it can be pushed forward by placing the fingers behind the angles of the lower jaw and pushing forwards. Maintaining the airway is always easier if the patient is nursed in an upright position or, if this is not feasible, in the lateral or tonsil position. The nurse should also watch for haemorrhage from the operation site. When the patient is fully conscious he should have a bowl into which saliva can drain. If there is any difficulty with speech, he should be given a pencil and pad and a foolproof way of attracting attention such as a bell or buzzer, checked to ensure it is in working order. Gentle moistening of the lips with cotton wool can also be a great comfort. Frequent mouth washes are essential, and should be given when the patient is sitting up.

If oral feeding is permitted, the diet must be a fluid one. A full nutritious diet can be given in a completely fluid form. If the ward has its own liquidiser, this is the best way to achieve a good, fluid

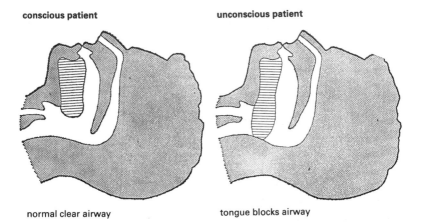

conscious patient   **unconscious patient**

normal clear airway   tongue blocks airway

Figure 13 How the airway of an unconscious patient can become blocked by the tongue

diet. Alternatively, the diet kitchen will be able to prepare meals for you. Oral feeding is sometimes not possible, and the patient will have a *nasogastric* tube (see Figure 23) inserted through the nose and into the stomach. This tube can become blocked and this is dangerous because fluid can regurgitate back into the throat and get into the lungs, causing an inhalation pneumonia. Before feeding via this tube, the nurse should ensure that the tube is sited correctly in the stomach. There are two ways of doing this: (1) aspirate some of the gastric content, and test the aspirate with a suitable reagent to determine its pH. The reaction should be acid: (2) Inject a small amount of air into the nasogastric tube, and simultaneously listen with a stethoscope over the epigastric region. If movement of gas in the stomach is heard to coincide with the injection of air by syringe the tube is in the stomach.

If there is still doubt about the position of the tube or if the patient shows any signs of cyanosis or respiratory distress, ask someone more experienced to check the tube for you. It may be necessary to pass the tube again, and even to check the position by taking an X-ray. It is most important that the principles of feeding via the nasogastric route are understood before this procedure is undertaken. If a nurse is unsure she should consult with a more senior colleague, or refer to more detailed literature. It is most important that the procedure is done correctly. A tube in the throat is never comfortable for the patient and frequently causes depression. The nurse should explain that it is only a temporary inconvenience to help his mouth heal more quickly and that soon he will be swallowing normally.

After the operation there may be quite severe pain which will require strong analgesics and sedatives. The most serious complication that can occur is *post-operative parotitis* or inflammation of the parotid salivary glands. This can occur after any operation, especially in elderly patients, but it is a direct reflection of poor nursing care and is far easier to prevent than to treat. The condition can be fatal, because infection easily spreads down into the lungs and causes a very virulent form of pneumonia. Infection can also spread into the oesophagus so that swallowing, even of fluids, is painful.

Diseases of the salivary glands

The parotid and submandibular glands are the largest and most important of the salivary glands. The three most important diseases to which they are prone are acute inflammation, the formation of calculi (stones) and tumours.

Acute inflammation

This is much more common in the parotid glands than in the submandibular glands. Infection can creep up the duct from a dry mouth and into the gland substance. The face is tender and swollen over the affected gland, and opening the mouth causes acute pain. An abscess may develop in the gland, and pus may be seen coming from the opening of the duct in the mouth. Treatment of the established condition may mean incision into the parotid gland to drain an abscess. Specimens of pus will be sent to the laboratory to identify the causative organism and to test its sensitivity to various antibiotics. Again, the need for oral hygiene is extremely important.

In children and rarely in adults, *both* parotid glands may become swollen and painful without any obvious sign of infection. This is *mumps*, a virus infection and an entirely separate condition.

Salivary gland calculi

Stones can form in the parotid and submandibular salivary glands. They do not occur in the normal gland but, if there is obstruction to the outflow of the saliva, either in the gland itself or in its duct, stagnation of the secretion occurs, and this is inevitably followed by infection. The solid matter or salts in the saliva are then deposited out of solution and a tiny stone is formed. Gradually the stone or *calculus* gets larger and causes symptoms. They are more common in the submandibular glands because their secretion is rather thick and contains mucus, whereas the parotid-gland secretion is thin and watery and therefore flows more easily. In addition, the parotid duct is straight and runs downwards across the cheek, while the submandibular duct runs a tortuous course and the saliva has to flow upwards into the floor of the mouth. It is not surprising, therefore, that 95 per cent of salivary calculi are formed in the submandibular gland.

The main symptom of these calculi is pain in the region of the affected gland. The patient notices that a swelling appears in the submandibular region at meal times but diminishes in size between meals. This is because the presence of food in the mouth stimulates the flow of saliva, which cannot get out because the duct is obstructed. The saliva is dammed back and the gland swells, and the rising tension within the gland is responsible for the pain.

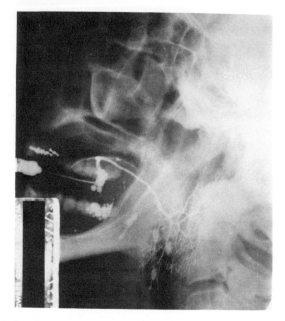

Figure 14 A parotid sialogram showing the main ducts of the parotid gland outlined with dye via a syringe and cannula

The enlarged gland can easily be felt. The only investigation necessary is an X-ray to prove the presence of a calculus. Occasionally a special X-ray called a *sialogram* is taken to show more clearly the interior of the gland. In this, a minute quantity of dye is injected into the duct, a picture is taken and all the branches of the ducts can be seen filled with dye (Figure 14). If left untreated, an abscess may develop within the gland because of the associated infection. All the usual signs of inflammation will then be present.

Treatment

The aim of the treatment is to remove the cause of obstruction. If the calculus can be felt near the duct orifice, the orifice is simply dilated and the calculus removed. If, however, the calculus is deep within the gland or if the gland has been damaged by repeated infection, it is better to effect a permanent cure by excising the gland.

The parotid gland may also become swollen at meal times if the duct orifice becomes narrowed or strictured. In this case, the doctor will dilate the orifice using *lachrymal probes*. This may be done under a local anaesthetic.

Tumours of the salivary glands

These are not common. The most important one is the mixed parotid tumour, so called because it contains several types of cells. It appears as a painless swelling in front of the ear. It enlarges very slowly and may have been present for many years before the patient seeks medical advice. However, it can become malignant if left untreated for long. The parotid gland consists of two lobes, a superficial lobe and a deep one. These tumours occur in the superficial lobe. Between these two lobes runs the facial nerve, which innervates all the facial muscles of expression. If the patient shows signs of weakness of the facial muscles or if the tumour becomes painful, malignant change in the tumour has probably already occurred. The correct treatment, therefore, is to excise all the superficial lobe containing the tumour before the malignant change takes place. Great care is taken not to damage the facial nerve, otherwise great disfigurement of the face may occur. This is the most important complication of the operation. It is vital therefore for the nurse to explain to the patient beforehand the nature of the operation and the risks involved. Explanation and information are vital for every patient, so that they may be aware of the options open to them, and can give informed consent to any treatment suggested. Alternatively, the patient may decide against treatment once he is in a position to make an informed choice.

A malignant tumour is treated by excising the whole of the parotid gland and removing the facial nerve, resulting in facial paralysis.

Post-operative nursing care

Following excision of the submandibular or parotid glands, blood and tissue fluids may collect in the space they occupied, a condition called *haematoma*. This haematoma may become infected and ruin the result of the operation. One way of avoiding this is to apply a pressure bandage as a figure-of-eight round the forehead and neck to obliterate the space. A better method is to employ a *suction drain* attached to a vacuum bottle to suck away the fluid as it collects. Before the wound is closed, an *atraumatic needle*, attached to the *drainage tube*, is guided into the tissues. The tube, which has the same diameter as the needle, is then joined to a vacuum bottle with a negative pressure of 600 mmHg (millimetres of mercury). At its exit point, the tube must be fixed with adhesive plaster, and the vacuum bottle changed when it is about two-thirds full. The nurse should observe the wound closely and ensure that the suction drain is working properly. Usually these drains have rubber 'antennae' which denote the presence or absence of a vacuum in the suction bottle. If such a vacuum is not indicated the nurse should look for possible causes, either in the drainage tube itself (which may have fallen out of the wound), or in a poor connection somewhere along the length of the tubing from the wound to the suction bottle. Any swelling should be reported immediately. Normally, because of the rich blood supply in the neck, these wounds heal quickly and the patient is able to leave hospital five days after the operation.

When caring for patients with disorders of the mouth the nurse needs to be very sensitive to the possible effects on the body image of the patient. The face and neck reflect, more than any other part of the anatomy, the personality of the individual. It may be most distressing for some patients to have any degree of disfigurement of this area, even if only temporary. Constant support and encouragement from the nurse is vital to the recovery and rehabilitation of the patient.

Four

The oesophagus

The *oesophagus* (the gullet) is a long muscular tube which runs from the back of the tongue through the chest, behind the trachea (windpipe) and the heart (Figure 15). It is simply a carrier of food and does not take any part in the digestive process. It enters the abdominal cavity through an opening in the diaphragm, called the *oesophageal hiatus*. It measures forty centimetres in length from the incisor teeth to the entrance of the stomach. The oesophagus passes through three regions of the body – the neck, where it is called the *cervical oesophagus*, the thorax, where it is called the *thoracic portion* of the oesophagus, and the abdomen, where it runs for two and a half centimetres inside the abdominal cavity before joining the stomach. The oesophagus, however, is not the straight tube that might be imagined. The upper part follows the curve of the neck

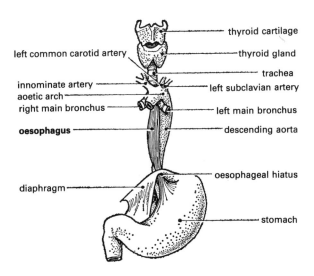

Figure 15 The oesophagus

and the lower part turns to the left before it enters the stomach. This information is important when instruments are passed into the oesophagus.

The entrance to the oesophagus is guarded by a circular muscle or sphincter. This is normally closed and opens only when we swallow. In a similar way the entrance to the stomach is guarded by a sphincter-like mechanism which prevents the reflux of gastric juice into the oesophagus.

When food has been swallowed, the muscles in the wall of the oesophagus propel it very rapidly downwards. At the same time, the sphincter mechanism at the lower end relaxes so that the food can enter the stomach. This is an active process and is under the control of the autonomic nervous system, transmitted via the vagus nerve. The food does not drop into the stomach by gravity alone. If this were so, it would be impossible to swallow a glass of water whilst standing on your head.

The oesophagus is lined by a thick epithelium called *squamous epithelium*. This is several layers thick in order to stand up to the wear and tear of different foods passing over it. It has nerve endings sensitive to hot, cold and stretch stimuli, so that swallowing a very hot liquid leads to a burning sensation in the oesophagus. If acid from the stomach comes in contact with the lining of the oeso-phagus, a burning sensation behind the sternum or breastbone (called heart-burn) is the result.

A knowledge of the exact position of the oesophagus in the chest and its relationship to neighbouring organs is very helpful in understanding the complications that can occur if the oesophagus is injured or diseased. The space in the centre of the chest between the two lungs is called the *mediastinum*. It is bounded by the sternum in front and the vertebral column behind, and runs from the thoracic inlet above to the diaphragm below. This space contains the heart and its great vessels, the trachea, oesophagus, thymus, lymph nodes and other structures and tissues. The oeso-phagus occupies the posterior portion of the mediastinum. The pericardium of the heart lies in front, and on either side is the covering membrane of the lungs (the pleura). The descending portion of the aorta (the main artery of the body) also runs down in the posterior mediastinum alongside the oesophagus. The other important structure in the posterior mediastinum is the thoracic duct, or main lymph duct. This carries the lymph from the abdomen up into the root of the neck, where it will discharge into the great veins on the left side. All these structures are loosely bound together with connective tissue.

Dysphagia

Dysphagia (difficulty in swallowing) is the most important symptom of oesophageal disease and is always treated as significant because it may be the only symptom of serious oesophageal disease. Furthermore, when it occurs, the disease may be already well advanced. If the oesophagus is completely obstructed due to disease, food will be regurgitated and the patient will progressively lose weight. If, for example, the sphincter mechanism at the lower end of the oesophagus becomes weakened, gastric juice will reflux into the lower end of the gullet causing *heartburn*. The lumen of the oesophagus may have become very narrow before the patient complains of dysphagia. This means that serious disease such as malignant growths can be well advanced before the first symptom occurs.

Investigation of dysphagia

A history of the patient is the doctor's first step in investigation. As cancer of the oesophagus is the most serious condition, a good doctor will want to rule this out before progressing further. Having elucidated all the facts about the dysphagia from the patient, the next step is to take an X-ray of the oesophagus. Because the oesophagus will not show up on an ordinary X-ray, the patient is given a barium-containing radio-opaque fluid to swallow. This is called a *barium swallow*, and enables the outline of the whole length of the oesophagus to be seen on the X-ray (Figure 16). Any obstruction or narrowing will then show up clearly.

The doctor's next step is to look directly into the oesophagus using an instrument called an *oesophagoscope*; the investigation is called an *oesophagoscopy*. This is the most important investigation of dysphagia and is always carried out, even if the barium swallow shows no abnormalities. Oesophagoscopy may be carried out by means of a rigid oesophagoscope (Figure 17) or the more modern and safer flexible fiberoptic instrument (Figure 18). The rigid oesophagoscope is a straight, hollow tube, forty centimetres long, usually made of brass. Lights inserted into the proximal end of the tube provide good illumination. A rigid oesophagoscopy is a major undertaking and, if not carried out expertly, can result in the death of the patient.

A general anaesthetic with full muscle relaxation is essential before rigid oesophagoscopy. Oesophagoscopy is easier to perform if the patient has a long mobile neck with small teeth. This is

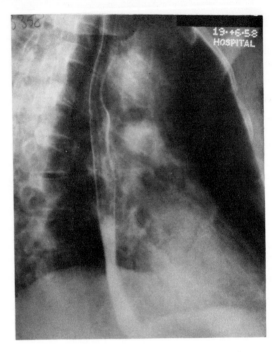

Figure 16 The X-ray appearance of a normal barium swallow

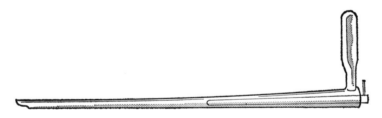

Figure 17 An oesophagoscope

because the neck must be fully extended in order to view the lower reaches of the oesophagus. In older people, the neck becomes more rigid, especially if there is arthritis in the cervical region of the spine; so, the older the patient, the more potentially dangerous is the investigation. In young people the chief difficulties encountered are the short 'bull-like' neck and the presence of large prominent teeth which make it difficult to pass the instrument into the oesophagus.

When the oesophagoscope has been passed successfully into the oesophagus, it is advanced gently until the obstruction comes into

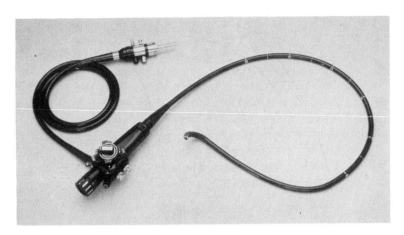

Figure 18 A flexible fiberoptic oesophago-gastroscope

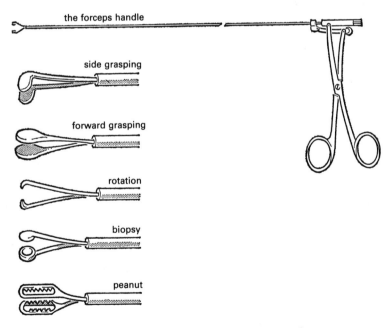

Figure 19 Different types of forceps for use with an oesophagoscope

view. The doctor can usually diagnose whether a lesion is benign or malignant simply by looking at it, but the final diagnosis is always made by taking a piece of tissue from the diseased area with long *biopsy forceps* (Fig. 19) introduced through the lumen of the oesophagoscope. This is sent to the laboratory for examination under the microscope.

By comparison, flexible fiberoptic oesophagoscopy can be carried out under intravenous valium following suitable premedication. This method has now almost superseded the rigid instrument. As with all investigations, the nurse should ensure that the patient has understood the explanation of the procedure before it takes place. Although an adequate explanation may have been given by a doctor or a nurse, the patient's anxiety about other matters may have prevented communication being effective. An easy way to check that the patient has understood, is to ask him to tell you what he thinks is about to happen to him.

Complications of oesophagoscopy

The most important complication that can arise from oesophagoscopy is perforation of the oesophagus. This can lead to death if it is not diagnosed and treated promptly, because infection always follows perforation and will spread into the posterior mediastinum causing serious illness. If a patient with a mere pinhole perforation of the oesophagus is given anything to eat or drink, his chances of recovery are seriously jeopardized.

The other, less serious, complications of the procedure include bruising of the lips and tongue from pressure of the instrument, chipping of prominent teeth and dislodging of loose ones. If the latter is not noticed at completion of the oesophagoscopy, the tooth may be swallowed or inhaled into the lungs, with subsequent development of a lung abscess.

Pre-operative nursing care

The nurse should check the state of the patient's mouth, including dentures, before the operation. This will provide a base-line for comparison in the event of any injury caused by the procedure. Such injury is rare, particularly with fiberoptic instruments, but damage to teeth, and trauma to the oral cavity, can occur with a rigid oesophagoscope. Before and after the operation, clear instructions should be given to the patient about refraining from drinking at all until he is specifically instructed to do so. An explanation should always be given: in this case, that the local anaesthetic used on the throat will upset the usual mechanism to prevent fluids passing to the lungs instead of to the oesophagus.

Post-operative nursing care

Following oesophagoscopy, observations of temperature, pulse
blood pressure, should be commenced immediately, and continued
regularly for eight hours initially, and then as the condition
dictates. This is to check for trauma and bleeding of the oesophageal wall, or for perforation. Observation also means looking at the
patient to detect visible signs of shock. There will be some soreness
of the throat, particular if a rigid oesophagoscope has been used,
but excessive soreness and increased dysphagia following this
procedure should be reported immediately.

Two further methods are sometimes used to solve the more
difficult cases of dysphagia. These are cineradiography, in which
the movements of the oesophagus are studied, and pressure-
recording, in which abnormalities of muscle contraction are investigated. Both are carried out in specialized hospital departments.

Several common disorders can affect the oesophagus.

Foreign bodies

Many different objects can be swallowed and become impacted in
the oesophagus. Children and patients with mental disorders
commonly swallow coins. Adults, particularly those without teeth,
can swallow pieces of meat or fish whose bones become lodged in
the gullet. Occasionally people swallow their dental plates. The
most serious complication is perforation of the oesophagus which
can arise if the swallowed object (e.g. a pin) has sharp or pointed
edges. If perforation occurs, infection will spread throughout the
mediastinum and death will result unless urgent operation is undertaken. The diagnosis is easily made. The patient will relate that he
has swallowed a foreign body, an event followed by pain and
difficulty in swallowing. Careful X-ray examination will show the
foreign body if it is radio-opaque. Sometimes a barium swallow may
be necessary.

Treatment

If a foreign body has been swallowed, it is most important that
nothing further is given by mouth until the object has been
removed. The act of swallowing stimulates contraction of the
muscle and may cause perforation of the wall.

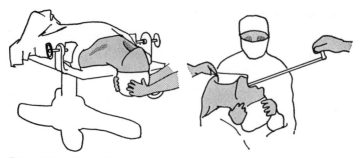

The position of the patient
on the operating table

The introduction of the oesophagoscope:
first stage, up to the circopharyngeus

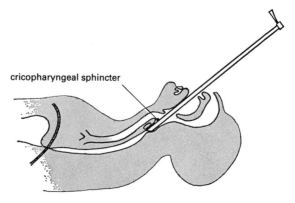

cricopharyngeal sphincter

Passing the circopharyngeus

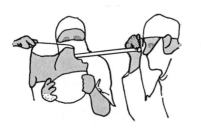

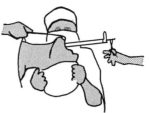

The oesophagoscope is advanced slowly
within the upper oesophagus

The foreign body has been visualized and is
grasped with alligator forceps

Figure 20 Oesophagoscopy

The object is usually removed with an oesophagoscope (Figure 20). Coins are usually easy to remove using a special instrument called a coin catcher. If the object is impacted solidly in the wall of the oesophagus, it ma be necessary to open the chest – a major operation – and remove it surgically.

Post-operative treatment

This is basically the same as that following any oesophagoscopy. If the foreign body was lodged for several days before oesophagoscopy was carried out, the lining of the oesophagus will be inflamed. The patient should not have any solid food for at least five days. A careful check on the patient's pulse and temperature during this time will enable the nurse to detect the warning signs of complications.

Oesophagitis

Oesophagitis (inflammation of the oesophageal lining) is perhaps the most common abnormal condition of the oesophagus. The usual cause is reflux of acid from the stomach into the lower oesophagus. This can occur only if the muscles guarding the lower end of the oesophagus become weakened, allowing the stomach to bulge up into the chest through the hiatus (gap) in the diaphragm, a condition known as *hiatus hernia* (Figure 21). If this reflux is allowed to continue for many years, the lower oesophagus will

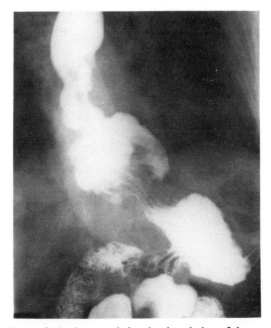

Figure 21 X-ray of a barium meal showing herniation of the stomach above the diaphragm in hiatus hernia

become so scarred that the lumen will become narrowed. The patient, who is most likely to be obese, complains of dysphagia because he has developed a *stricture* (narrowing) of the lower oesophagus. Other forms of oesophagitis can result from swallowing corrosive fluids; scarring will again result in a stricture, and increasing dysphagia is the main complaint. All cases of oesophagitis are investigated chiefly by oesophagoscopy and biopsy.

Hiatus hernia

Most pregnant women get a temporary hiatus hernia between the sixth and ninth months of pregnancy and complain bitterly of heartburn and regurgitation of acid fluid into the back of the throat. When the pregnancy is over, the symptoms disappear spontaneously because the pressure of the enlarged uterus on the stomach has been relieved. Other cases of hiatus hernia will usually require treatment.

Treatment

All cases are treated medically in the first instance. The principles of treatment are:

(a) weight reduction;

(b) the avoidance of all tight clothing such as corsets, since tight clothes increase the intra-abdominal pressure and increase the amount of reflux;

(c) avoidance of all unnecessary stooping and bending, since acid gastric juice will flow more easily into the oesophagus if aided by gravity;

(d) regular administration of drugs called *antacids*, which will help to neutralize the acid, relieve symptoms and minimize the damage to the oesophagus.

These simple measures are adequate in the majority of uncomplicated cases. If the patient cooperates, yet the symptoms persist, especially in young people, surgical treatment is indicated, the aims of which are to tighten the hiatus so that reflux may be prevented, and to reduce the amount of acid being secreted by the patient. This may involve a *gastrectomy* or *vagotomy* (see p. 69). The hiatus may be reached via the abdomen or the chest.

Complications

A hiatus hernia can produce a severe degree of *anaemia*, due to the bleeding of the inflamed oesophagus. Viewed through an oesophagoscope, the lining or *mucosa* of the oesophagus appears fiery red and bleeds readily when touched. This also happens when food passes over it. Over a long period of time small, but repeated, losses of blood occur, with the development of a typical iron-deficiency anaemia. The patient does not know he is losing blood, as he cannot see it. If the stools are examined for blood, the test will be positive. This is an example of *occult bleeding* from the alimentary tract. In some patients, therefore, the presenting symptoms may result from the anaemia, and its cause should be thoroughly investigated before the anaemia itself is treated.

A typical *gastric ulcer* may develop in the oesophagus of a patient with a hiatus hernia (Figure 22). This is not as strange as it seems, because the normal oesophagus has no protection against the acid made in the stomach. If the reflux of acid-containing fluid continues, the oesophageal mucosa may become so eroded that an active ulcer crater develops.

If a *peptic stricture* (a stricture caused by peptic secretions) has resulted from the hiatus hernia, the narrowed portion of the oesophagus may have to be excised. This is an extremely difficult operation, and a hiatus hernia should not reach this condition untreated.

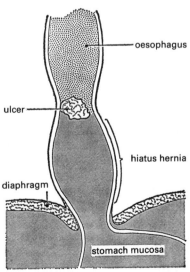

Figure 22 Ulceration with hiatus hernia

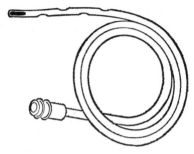

Figure 23 A nasogastric tube

Pre-operative nursing care

Every patient who undergoes surgical treatment should have a nasogastric tube passed into the stomach before the operation. A nasogastric tube (Figure 23) is a long plastic tube which is passed slowly and carefully into the patient's nose, down his throat and into his stomach. It is much easier to do this if the patient is sitting up and cooperating than if he is fully anaesthetized. Following insertion, the same tests can be used as described in Chapter 3, for ascertaining the correct position of the tube. Aspiration of stomach gas and secretions, will be necessary until the patient's bowel has resumed normal function.

Post-operative care

As for all abdominal or thoracic operations, the patient should be actively encouraged by the nurse to perform the breathing exercises he has learnt from the physiotherapist, as, without encouragement, the patient may be reluctant to do these exercises. Altering the intra-thoracic pressure, and therefore the intra-abdominal pressure, will put stress onto the wound-site, and the patient may feel that it is about to burst open. The best way to overcome these fears is for the nurse to stay with the patient initially as he does his exercises so that he can be reassured that nothing will go wrong.

For patients on bedrest, leg exercises to prevent circulatory stasis should also be regularly performed. Failure to do so will increase the risk of deep-vein thrombosis in their legs, which may in itself lead to pulmonary embolism and collapse. It is generally acceptable for patients to suck ice, or take sips of water (not exceeding 30 ml/ hour) orally, whilst the nasogastric tube is in place. It is a pleasant feeling for the patient, and can usually be aspirated back via the nasogastric tube. At least it creates a refreshing feeling in the mouth.

However, there may be contra-indications to this, so it is always wise for the nurse to check the surgeon's notes for any specific instructions, or ask someone more senior if she is not sure.

Benign strictures of the oesophagus

Benign strictures, other than peptic strictures, may be the result of scarring following damage to the oesophagus wall by a foreign body or as a result of swallowing corrosive fluids. Not uncommonly a stricture results from inhaling hot fumes. A patient may be admitted to hospital with severe burns of the face and lips as a result of coming into contact with hot explosive fumes. The burned face will receive expert treatment, and the patient will make an excellent recovery. Months later he may complain of dysphagia and investigations will reveal a stricture of the oesophagus. When the patient was burned, he inhaled and swallowed hot gases which inflamed his oesophagus. The scars in the oesophagus subsequently caused a stricture.

In a similar way, if a nasogastric tube is kept in position for many weeks, without giving the patient anything to drink normally, it can act as an irritant. Inflammation will then be followed by a stricture. This should not be allowed to happen, and patients should drink 'around the tube' whenever possible.

Symptoms

Increasing dysphagia is the only complaint associated with a benign stricture of the oesophagus. There are no signs.

Treatment

Simple strictures are treated by gradual dilatation with *bougies*. A bougie is a slender, tapered rod usually made of gum elastic (Figure 24). Using an oesophagoscope, graduated sizes are inserted through the stricture to stretch it. A peptic stricture cannot be treated in

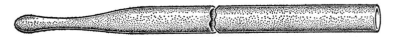

Figure 24 A bougie; it is made of gum elastic and is about 63 cm long

this way because it normally causes more acid to be refluxed into the oesophagus, and the result would be an even longer stricture.

Post-operative nursing care

This is similar to that following the removal of a foreign body.

Malignant strictures of the oesophagus

Caricinoma of the oesophagus is a very serious condition (Figure 25). Unless treated, dysphagia becomes so severe that the patient is unable to swallow even his own saliva, and will starve to death. Increasing dysphagia and progressive weight loss are the commonest symptoms. Food is difficult to swallow at first and later becomes impossible. With time, even liquids are swallowed only with the greatest difficulty. When the patient is admitted to hospital, he may be emaciated and dehydrated. In addition, the cancer may have spread outside the oesophagus and invaded neighbouring organs, leading to a variety of symptoms. The oesophagus above the growth usually becomes dilated and food may remain in

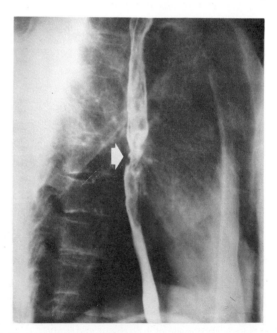

Figure 25 X-ray appearance of carcinoma of the oesophagus

this dilated portion for many days, leading to pressure on the important structures in the posterior mediastinum. As the patient tries to eat more, the oesophagus will overflow and foul-smelling stagnant fluid will be regurgitated. If this fluid spills over into the trachea, especially when the patient is lying flat in bed at night, it may cause an *inhalation pneumonia*. This is invariably fatal and is a not uncommon mode of death in the untreated case.

The diagnosis is made by the investigations described above.

Treatment

The most desirable treatment is to remove the oesophagus (oesophagectomy). It is a very severe operation, as the oesophagus is so deeply placed in the chest. Furthermore, some form of new oesophagus must be fashioned to bridge the gap – for this, the stomach, small intestine or colon may be used. Thus, both the chest and the abdomen must be opened.

Some growths in the oesophagus can be reduced in size by radiotherapy. In very elderly, unfit patients, for whom major surgery is not possible, radiotherapy can cause a regression of the tumour. More commonly, however, it is used to kill off any residual tumour following surgery. Radiotherapy can be a very distressing experi-

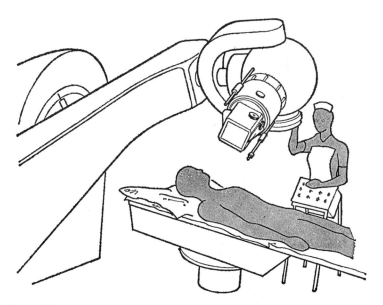

Figure 26 A cobalt treatment room. Radioactive carbon-60 is used in deep ray treatment for certain cancers

ence for the patient. Organs adjacent to the tumour, such as the lung, will inevitably receive some irradiation. Painful blistering of the overlying skin was once a further common complication but, with the modern supervoltage machines, such as the cobalt unit (Figure 26), this has been reduced to a minimum. Nausea, loss of appetite and depression are common, and the patient will undoubtedly need a great deal of reassurance.

Pre-operative nursing care

A patient who is to undergo major surgery to the oesophagus should be in the best possible condition for his body to deal with this intervention. If symptoms have been present for some time, he may well be anaemic, nutritionally deficient and have suffered considerable weight loss. An intensive nutrition programme, including vitamins and iron as required, should then be planned pre-operatively. The nurse can do much to ensure that such a programme is effectively completed. Occasionally, intravenous feeding may be necessary if absorption from the gut is poor or an obstruction is present. During this delay before surgery, the time can be well spent in allowing the patient and relatives to adjust gradually to the fact of surgery. More time can be taken to deal with queries and talk things through with the patient. If the patient is on bedrest, constant care of the skin must also be undertaken to prevent pressure sores developing. Broken areas and poorly nourished skin and tissue will produce a potentially infectious focus, and could delay planned surgery. Mouth care is also vital, particularly if little oral fluid is tolerated.

Post-operative care

Post-operatively, an intravenous infusion will continue, initially with blood and fluid to replace losses at surgery, and subsequently for nutrition again. The nasogastric tube will also remain, to allow aspiration of fluid and escape of gas as previously described.

As the thorax will have been surgically opened – a thoracotomy – there will also be an under-water-seal drainage tube in situ (or more than one) to drain air and fluid from the pleural cavity, to allow normal expansion of the lung. (The pleural cavity is normally only a potential cavity. If it contains air or fluid, it will compromise lung function, preventing normal expansion.) These tubes will be removed when drainage is complete and internal healing has restored normal function.

Observation of the patient's general condition should be carefully monitored. This includes regular observation, by looking at the patient and noting the signs of shock, infection or haemorrhage, as well as the recording of temperature, pulse, blood pressure *and* respirations. Accurate fluid balance is vital (see Chapter 2), particularly if the patient is elderly when overloading of their circulation can cause extra strain on the heart and precipitate cardiac failure and hypertension. Gradual mobilisation of the patient can commence, with support and encouragement, and as drainage tubes are removed and the shock of surgery resolved, this can be increased from sitting in a chair by the bed, to short walks around the ward and to the toilet.

On the fifth post-operative day, a gastrografin swallow may be performed in the x-ray department (Fig. 27) to check healing of the new oesophagus. If satisfactory, oral fluids may be commenced gradually and increased with removal of the nasogastric tube. The exact timing varies for each individual patient, and specific instructions should be sought in each case. Fluids only are taken until the 10th to **14th day post-operatively.**

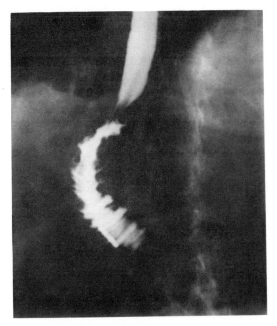

Figure 27 **X-ray appearance of a gastrografin swallow taken on the fifth** post-operative day following total gastrectomy. The anastomosis between the oesophagus and small intestine has healed. The nasogastric tube is still in position

As this is a major operation, complications can and do arise, and the nurse can be the first to note them and prevent them from getting worse. Chest infections, wound infections or breakdown, haemorrhage or surgical emphysema can occur. The latter is a swelling of tissue, particularly in the neck, due to air escaping from the lungs and lodging there: the signs are crackling on palpation and dyspnoea.

Palliative operations for carcinoma of the oesophagus

Carcinoma of the oesophagus is frequently found to be too far advanced to cure by surgical means and, in this case, the doctor may decide on a palliative operation (one to reduce the severity of the disease). Dysphagia is a most distressing symptom and an attempt is made to relieve it so that the patient will spend his remaining days in comfort. A patient who continually drools saliva out of his mouth because he cannot swallow is in a pitiful state, and the best palliation can be achieved by a by-pass operation. The stomach or a loop of small intestine is joined to the side of the oesophagus above the growth, although this is a very serious undertaking in patients who are old, ill and weak.

It may be simpler to dilate the malignant stricture under general anaesthetic and insert a tube through the narrowed portion of the oesophagus. An example of a modern tube is the Mousseau-Barbin tube (Figure 28). This has a funnel-shaped upper end which sits on top of the stricture, and a tapered lower end which can be guided into the stomach.

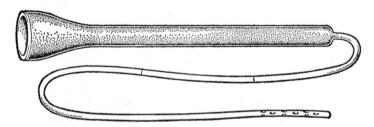

Figure 28 A Mousseau–Barbin tube

Post-operative nursing care

A patient undergoing such a palliative operation will still be debilitated, and will need much encouragement to have the will to recover. More practically, the nurse needs to ensure that further distress is not caused by her negligence to keep the tube patent by washing it through with fizzy drinks, e.g. soda-water, lemonade, or tonic water, after each meal. Tougher, larger pieces of food should be minced or even liquidised. However, it is important to try and retain the individual components of the meal, so that they are at least recognisable by colour. In this way, eating meals can be as normal as circumstances will allow.

Radiotherapy has an important part to play in palliation. Once the patient can swallow, and provided the growth is radiosensitive, the patient will probably benefit from shrinkage of the tumour through radiotherapy.

Rarer causes of dysphagia

Pharyngeal pouches

These are sac-like protrusions from the lining of the extreme upper end of the oesophagus and occur typically in elderly people (Figure 29). Food gets trapped in the pouch instead of being swallowed, and patients complain of food sticking in the throat; they also lose weight. Treatment is by excision of the pouch.

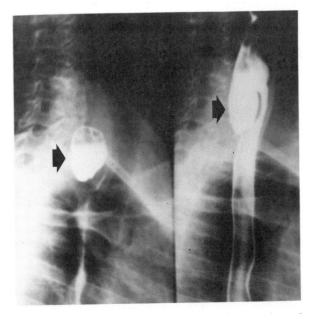

Figure 29 An X-ray showing barium held up in a pharyngeal pouch

Achalasia of the cardia

The *cardia* is the junction between the oesophagus and the stomach. In this complaint, the smooth muscle at the lower end of the oesophagus remains tightly shut instead of relaxing during swallowing. As a result, the *bolus* (ball) of food is held up. In an effort to overcome this difficulty, the wall of the oesophagus above this area hypertrophies and the oesophagus becomes dilated. Patients experience great discomfort in swallowing and, in severe cases, regurgitation of food occurs. These symptoms may take years to develop, so it may be some time before the patient seeks relief. A barium swallow gives a very characteristic picture (Figure 30) but, in all cases, oesophagoscopy is essential. The chief complication of achalasia, apart from malnutrition, is regurgitation of food into the lungs – with the attendant danger of inhalation pneumonia.

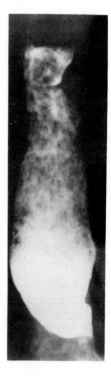

Figure 30 X-ray picture of a barium swallow, showing achalasia of the cardia. The lower part of the oesophagus is tightly shut, while the upper part is dilated and full of retained food

Treatment

The principle of treatment is to get the muscle at the lower end of the oesophagus to relax. This can be achieved in several ways.

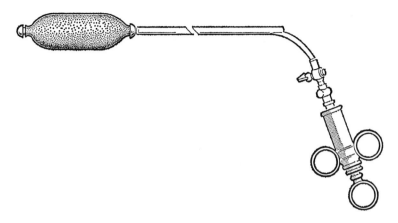

Figure 31 The Negus hydrostatic bag

Antispasmodic drugs give temporary relief in early cases. Alternatively, the lower end of the oesophagus may be stretched using a special instrument called a *Negus hydrostatic bag* (Figure 31). This is introduced via an oesophagoscope, and when the bag is in the lower end of the oesophagus, it is distended with water. This forcibly stretches the muscle so that food can now be swallowed. The chief danger of this form of treatment is the risk of perforation of the oesophagus. As it involves some risk to the patient, it should not be carried out more than twice. If symptoms recur, the third form of treatment, Heller's operation, may be preferable. This operation involves division of the muscle at the lower end of the oesophagus down to the mucous membrane. It is similar to Rammstedt's operation for infantile pyloric stenosis, which is discussed in the next chapter (see p. 66).

Pre-operative nursing care

If retention oesophagitis is present, the most important duty is to carry out oesophageal lavage to empty the oesophagus.

Post-operative nursing care

Afterwards, because the main complication of the operation is inadvertent opening of the oesophageal mucosa, the nurse should watch closely for signs of mediastinitis. The nursing care is similar to that described above.

Haemorrhage from the oesophagus

The most important cause of severe haemorrhage from the oesophagus is *oesophageal varices* – varicose veins at the lower end of the
oesophagus (Figure 32). All the venous blood from the alimentary
tract is returned to the liver via the portal vein. The blood is detoxi-
cated in the liver and then drains into the *inferior vena cava* via the
hepatic veins at the back of the liver. From here, it enters the right
chambers of the heart. If there is any obstruction to the flow of
blood in the liver (as would occur in *cirrhosis* of the liver), the blood
by-passes the liver via a system of veins behind the stomach. These
commanicate with the veins in the oesophagus and drain into the
vena cava and so to the heart. These veins are thin-walled and small
and, in order to accommodate the increased volume of blood trav-
elling along the by-pass, they become enlarged, tortuous and
dilated, and oesophageal varices are formed. Because their walls are
thin and covered only by mucous membrane, and because the blood
is flowing at an abnormally high pressure, these veins are liable to
rupture, with resultant massive **haemorrhage.**

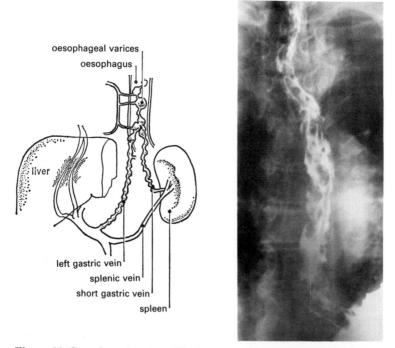

Figure 32 Oesophageal varices. The **barium swallow X-ray shows multiple**
filling defects caused by the varices

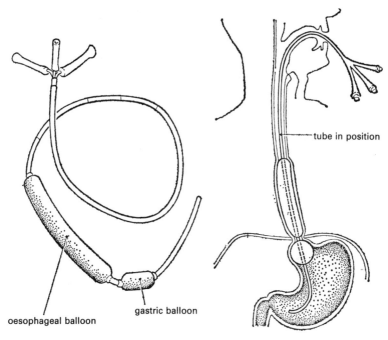

Figure 33 A Sengstaken tube and balloon

Treatment

Emergency treatment aims to control the haemorrhage and make
certain that the blood in the alimentary tract is evacuated as quickly
as possible. A *Sengstaken tube* is passed to control the haemorrhage.
This is a rubber tube with an outer cuff which, when inflated,
applies pressure to the bleeding vessels (Figure 33). The patient
may be fed through the central lumen.

Post-operative nursing care

Whilst the cuff is blown up, the patient will be unable to take fluid
via the tube, or orally. The nurse should regularly check the
position of the tube, and ensure that it has not slipped up the
oesophagus where the inflated cuff could cause problems to the
airway. Before feeding, the same checks should be made as with
any nasogastric tube (see above).

Blood is evacuated from the alimentary tract with daily or twice-
daily *colonic washouts* until the return shows that all old blood has
been removed. If blood is left in the colon, the poisonous products

which the liver cannot deal with accumulate, and coma results.

When the immediate emergency is over, plans are made to prevent a recurrence of haemorrhage. This will mean making a permanent opening between the portal vein and the inferior vena cava. By this means blood will be shunted away from the dangerous oesophageal veins. This will be discussed further in relation to diseases of the liver.

Five
The stomach and duodenum

The stomach is a flask-shaped bag which lies transversely in the upper part of the abdomen (Figure 34 and 35). Its main function is to convert solid food into a fluid of porridge-like consistency and to propel it, in a controlled manner, into the duodenum. To digest the food, the stomach secretes 2000–3000 ml of gastric juice every day. The digestion process works automatically once the food enters the stomach.

The stomach wall consists of three layers of muscles, longitudinal, circular and oblique (Figure 36), and these are concerned with the movements of propulsion, churning and mixing of food. The food particles must be brought into close contact with the gastric juice, so the churning movement is very important. Whilst the food is being mixed in the stomach, the pylorus remains tightly shut, aided by the circular layer of muscle. When the food is converted to a fluid-like consistency (*chyme*), the pylorus relaxes and the fluid is squirted into the duodenum, aided by the longitudinal muscle layer.

Both these sets of muscles are under the control of the automatic nervous system and mediated by a specific nerve (the *vagus nerve*) which travels down on the wall of the oesophagus and enters the abdomen through the opening in the diaphragm called the *oesophageal hiatus*. It then sends branches to all parts of the stomach. When this nerve is stimulated, the stomach muscles contract, i.e. it is the *motor nerve* of the stomach. The vagus also stimulates the gastric glands of the lining of the stomach to secrete hydrochloric acid; so, if this nerve is cut or fails to work, the stomach will be paralysed and fluid will stagnate in it. Furthermore the acid output of the stomach will be reduced. The gastric juice is made in the stomach lining (the *mucous membrane*) from the blood circulating through it. The mucous membrane has a very large surface area and is made up of many folds (*gastric folds*). It is salmon-pink in colour, but its thickness and appearance vary in the three parts of the

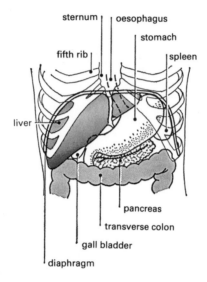

Figure 34 The stomach in the abdominal cavity

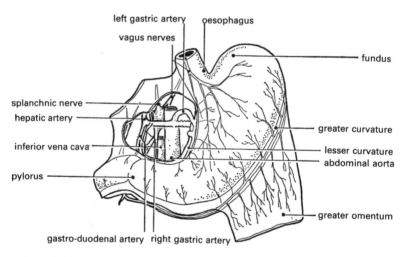

Figure 35 The anatomy of the stomach

stomach. In the fundus and body, it is quite thick and the folds are high, and most of the gastric juice is produced here. In the antrum it is much thinner, and here the hormone *gastrin* is manufactured.

In order to secrete 3000 ml of gastric juice every day, the stomach needs a very rich blood supply. The arteries encircle the stomach from one main source (the *coeliax axis*) via branches called the left

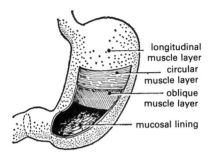

Figure 36 The stomach wall

and right *gastric arteries* on the lesser curve and the left and right *gastroepiploic arteries* on the greater curve (Figure 37). The branches penetrate the muscle to form a fine network near the mucous membrane. From here the blood is returned by a system of veins to the portal vein (see p. 8) and from there to the liver. Following a meal the blood-flow through the stomach is very large, but when the stomach is empty little blood is required. The volume of blood is regulated by tiny nerves which accompany the arteries. These are the sympathetic nerves which dilate and constrict the arteries as the need arises.

There is sometimes a feeling of drowsiness after a meal. This is because the sympathetic nerves dilate the gastric arteries and blood is diverted to the stomach from the organs such as the limbs and

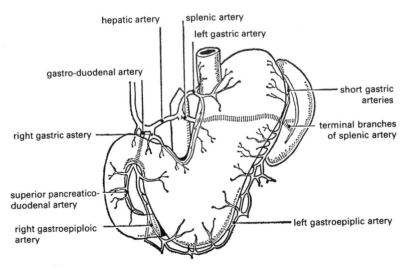

Figure 37 The blood supply to the stomach

lungs. Consequently, less blood flows to the brain, which therefore receives less oxygen.

Gastric juice

The most important constituent of the gastric juice is *hydrochloric acid*, a very strong acid which would burn the skin if dropped on it. But the stomach lining is protected by a layer of mucus, so it is not damaged by this strong acid. The acid in the stomach is produced in a remarkable way. Each gastric gland is like a tube whose sides are lined by cells which produce *mucin*, a colourless sticky substance. At the bottom of the tube are the cells (the *parietal cells*) which produce the hydrochloric acid. When the gland is stimulated, the tube fills with a mixture of mucin and acid. The mucin is discharged first, forming the protective coating on the surface of the stomach, then the acid is discharged. In the early years of life, a lot of mucin is produced but, as the body ages, the gastric mucosa becomes thinner and the gastric glands shrivel (*atrophy*), producing less mucus. The acid is then far more likely to erode the mucosa and cause a *gastric ulcer*, which is why gastric ulcers are more common in elderly people than in young people. Other constituents of the gastric juice are the enzymes, especially pepsin.

Hunger provides the first stimulus for the secretion of gastric juices, then the appetizing smell of food triggers impulses in the vagus. These travel to the gastric glands and gastric juice is poured out in preparation for the reception of the food in the stomach. At this point the mucosa has become bright red, suffused with blood. When the appetite has been satisfied, the stimulation from the vagus nerve is switched off, but the stomach still requires gastric juice to complete the process of digestion. At this point the secondary stimulation is brought into play. The mere contact of food with the mucosa stimulates it to produce the hormone *gastrin*. This hormone circulates in the blood stream and, when it reaches the parietal cells, it stimulates them to produce more acid. This process continues until all the food is reduced to liquid *acid chyme*. The stomach then empties, and the mechanism is switched off.

There are several other ways in which the production of gastric juice may be stimulated. Perhaps the most common is worry or stress (causing 'butterflies' in the stomach). Alcohol is another potent stimulator, as is nicotine. Another substance which acts as a stimulator is *histamine*, which may be injected subcutaneously to stimulate the parietal cells. However, the parietal cells must be controlled, or they would produce too much acid and this would be harmful. So, for most of the time, only a proportion of the cells are working, while the others are resting. The resting cells can be brought into play whenever the need arises.

When the stomach is not functioning correctly, the main warning symptom is pain. However, pain is often difficult to describe accurately. If pain arises from the stomach or duodenum it is always felt in the *epigastrium* (the part of the abdominal wall between the *umbilicus* and *xiphisternum* – part of the breastbone) and it is usually related to the taking of food. Loss of appetite is another sign that something may be amiss. Vomiting is a third warning sign which may lead a person to consult the doctor.

Investigation of disorders

In investigations of disorders of the stomach, the doctor will first take an accurate history. This is very important as there may be no physical signs present. In cases of vomiting, the character and frequency and type of vomiting will be determined.

If the patient is admitted to hospital, three general investigations are always carried out. As before, careful explanation must be given to the patient, and basic understanding checked by the nurse. The three investigations are:

(a) haemoglobin estimation (the patient may look quite normal and yet may be anaemic);

(b) chest X-ray;

(c) urine analysis: this is carried out by the nurse, and it is important to discover if any sugar is present in the urine, particularly if an operation is planned.

Special investigations

Barium meal

If a solution of barium sulphate is swallowed and an X-ray picture is taken of the stomach, its size and outline can be seen. The normal stomach movements can be studied, and the rate at which the stomach empties can be recorded. Ulcers (Figure 38) and tumours of the stomach are seen as ulcer craters on the wall of the stomach or as a filling defect in the stomach. The nurse must ensure that the patient fasts for twelve hours beforehand.

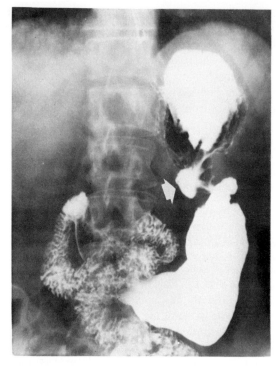

Figure 38 Barium meal X-ray showing a typical gastric ulcer

Gastroscopy

A gastroscope (or fibroscope) is a long flexible instrument through which the whole of the interior of the stomach can be visualized in the conscious patient (Figure 18). It is used to detect gastric ulcers or carcinomas of the stomach, or to take biopsies of suspicious-looking areas. Photographic records, either still or cine, can also be obtained.

The patient is always conscious since a general anaesthetic would stop the normal stomach movements taking place. Careful preparation of the patient for fibroscopy is essential. The main aspects of this are:

(a) The stomach should be empty. The patient should be given nothing to eat or drink for 12 hours beforehand (he should also be told not to accept any food from visitors).

(b) The patient should be given premedication to make him drowsy and to dry up secretions. *Omnopon* and *atropine* are suitable drugs and should be given about 1½ hours before the investigation (if they are given earlier their effect will have worn off and, if later, they will not take effect).

(c) The patient's throat should be anaesthetized to prevent gagging when the instrument is passed. The easiest method is for the nurse to give the patient half an anaesthetic lozenge at the time of premedication and the remainder about half an hour before the investigation. In nervous patients, 5–10 mg of *valium* may be given intravenously before the fibroscope is passed.

(d) The patient should not be allowed anything to eat or drink for four hours because firstly, the local anaesthetic to the throat affects the cough reflex and, secondly, it is essential to ensure that no trauma has occurred to the oesophageal or gastric mucosa. Regular pulse recordings should be made at least hourly for this period, and more frequently if the condition warrants it. The nurse must report any consistent change in pulse rate immediately. It may be a warning of haemorrhage or perforation.

Tests of acid secretion

An indication of the ability of the stomach to secrete hydrochloric acid is obviously important, for example, when investigating peptic ulcers. In the past, a *test meal* used to be given. Various meals (often gruel) were given, and then the stomach contents were aspirated and the acid content analysed. Later, the drug *histamine* was discovered to be a potent stimulator of hydrochloric acid secretion. A small dose of histamine was injected subcutaneously and, for the following hour, the stomach contents were aspirated and analysed.

It was found that the stomach was capable of secreting more acid than was originally thought. People with a duodenal ulcer secreted far more acid than those with a normal stomach, or even those with a gastric ulcer. It was also found that the more histamine that was injected, the more acid was secreted – up to a maximum dose, when no further increase in secretion occurred. This was called the maximal histamine test. If no acid at all is produced (i.e. the stomach is incapable of producing acid), the condition is known as *achlorhydria*.

It has now been found that gastrin is a more potent stimulator of acid secretion than histamine, although in the pure state it is very expensive since it has to be extracted from the antra of hogs' stomachs and then purified. However, it can now be synthesized artificially and can be mass-produced cheaply. Thus the maximum amount of acid any patient can produce can be accurately measured.

The commonest disorders of the stomach and duodenum involve ulcers, but pyloric stenosis and tumours are also common.

Congenital pyloric stenosis

This is a narrowing of the pylorus (outlet of the stomach) and is caused by a thickening of the circular muscle (sphincter) at the pylorus. However, it is not known why this occurs. The baby (very often a boy) is quite fit at birth, but after a few weeks begins to vomit, usually after a feed. Vomiting in very young babies is common but, in pyloric stenosis, the fluid spurts out in a jet from the baby's mouth. He may vomit feeds given a long time previously. The baby loses weight rapidly because of the loss of fluid and dehydration occurs, resulting in a wizened appearance.

The thickened pylorus may be most easily felt within the baby's abdomen just after a feed. Sometimes the outline of the stomach can be seen as it contracts strongly in an attempt to overcome the obstruction, a movement called *visible peristalsis*.

Mild cases may improve if the dehydration is corrected by giving intravenous saline (this replaces the fluid lost by vomiting). The child can also be given an antispasmodic drug (such as *eumydrin*), which may relax the pyloric sphincter. In this treatment the nurse must keep an accurate record of the amount of fluid given and the amount lost by vomiting.

If medical treatment is not successful, the surgeon will divide the thickened pyloric muscle down to the mucosa so that the stomach can empty readily (Figure 39). Any operation on a three-week-old

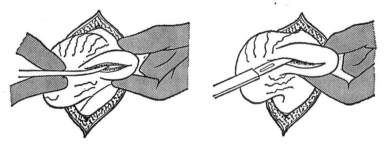

Figure 39 Rammstedt's operation for congenital pyloric stenosis. An incision is made in the long axis of the pylorus, taking care not to penetrate the mucosa; this should divide all but the deepest circular muscle fibres. The remaining fibres are then teased apart with a blunt dissector

baby is a serious undertaking. If the child is already weakened by dehydration, this must obviously be corrected beforehand by a scalp vein transfusion. The baby may be nursed in an incubator to provide a stable environment during this vulnerable period.

After the operation, very small amounts of *glucosaline* should be given at first, gradually increasing to normal milk-feeding. But the most important aspect of post-operative care is to guard against infection. These babies are particularly prone to gastro-enteritis. This condition can be fatal in one so young.

Peptic ulcers

A peptic ulcer is an ulcer that can occur in any part of the gastro-intestinal mucosa exposed to the action of gastric juice. They are most commonly found in the first part of the duodenum, when they are known as *duodenal ulcers*, and in the stomach, when they are known as *gastric ulcers*. If gastric juice refluxes into the oesophagus, a peptic ulcer may occur in the lower part.

Duodenal ulcers

The duodenal mucosa secretes an alkaline fluid and, unlike the mucosa of the stomach, has no protection against acid. If it is constantly subjected to high concentrations of acid, it is likely to become eroded and a duodenal ulcer may develop. The exact cause of duodenal ulceration is not known, but in the majority of cases it is certainly associated with an excessive production of acid by the stomach. When it is active it causes pain, especially when food is eaten, and this is the chief symptom.

Once a duodenal ulcer has developed, it remains for life, but its natural tendency is to heal up, leaving a scar in the duodenum. If, however, the stimulus to excessive acid production recurs, the scar tissue is likely to break down and ulcerate again. This is why symptoms of duodenal ulcer are *periodic*. A patient may remain symptom-free for months in which the ulcer is said to be *in remission*. But since smoking, worry, excessive alcohol, irregular meals and stress of any kind all stimulate acid secretion, if a patient with a duodenal ulcer is frequently subjected to these stimuli, his ulcer will recur. If this state of affairs is allowed to continue, one of the complications of duodenal ulcer will almost certainly occur.

If the ulcer is on the anterior wall of the duodenum, it may *perforate* and cause a general peritonitis (see p. 80). If it is on the posterior wall of the duodenum, the crater may erode the pancreas (see Figure 60). This usually causes pain in the back, which is why doctors always enquire about this symptom. The gastro-duodenal artery runs down between the duodenum and the head of the pancreas. The ulcer crater may erode this artery and cause a severe *haemorrhage*. If this blood is vomited up, it is referred to as a *haematemesis*. But, if the bleeding is slower, the blood will pass through the small bowel and colon and will be passed out through the rectum, a condition called *melaena*. The stools passed are a jet-black tarry colour because, when blood passes through the bowel, it is altered chemically to give it a characteristic black colour. This type of stool always implies bleeding high up in the alimentary tract. The most common cause is a peptic ulcer.

If there are two ulcers in the duodenum, one on the anterior wall and the second on the posterior wall and they heal and break down repeatedly, they may cause so much scar tissue (*fibrosis*) that the pyloric opening into the duodenum becomes narrowed, causing *pyloric stenosis* (see p. 66). The muscles in the wall of the stomach will get thicker (*hypertrophy*) in an attempt to overcome the obstruction and, when they cannot get any thicker, the stomach will dilate. A vicious circle has now developed – on the one hand, the food is in continual contact with the antrum and it cannot leave the stomach, so acid will continue to be secreted; on the other hand, this acid will keep the duodenal ulcer active and so it persists until the obstruction is relieved. Vomiting occurs, usually containing food eaten the previous day. (It may have an offensive smell because of the stagnation in the stomach.)

Duodenal ulcers never become malignant and in this respect differ dramatically from gastric ulcers, which may undergo malignant change.

Treatment

An uncomplicated ulcer is usually treated medically in the first instance. The aims are to ensure that the ulcer heals and to keep it healed for as long as possible. The first aim can be achieved by making sure that the patient has complete rest, diluting the acid content of the stomach with frequent meals and neutralizing the acid by alkalis and buffers, such as milk. Once the ulcer is healed, the best way to keep it healed is for the patient to eat regular meals. However, he should avoid those foods which he knows from experience cause discomfort. The patient should clearly understand that the alkalis should be taken as prescribed by the doctor (usually first thing in the morning, between meals and last thing at night – i.e. when the stomach is empty), and not merely when he is suffering from indigestion. All stimuli to acid production should be avoided as much as possible, the same applies to stress of any kind, alcohol or tobacco.

However, if complications occur, or the ulcer does not respond to careful medical treatment, surgical treatment may be necessary to permanently reduce the amount of acid secreted by the stomach. This can be achieved in two ways. Firstly, the nervous stimulation to acid production can be removed by cutting the vagus nerves; this is called a *vagotomy* (Figure 40).

If the main nerves are divided, not only are the branches to the stomach divided, but so also are the branches to the liver, gall bladder, pancreas and small intestine. This produces undesirable side-effects in a proportion of patients, of which the chief one is severe diarrhoea. Selective vagotomy is a modification of this operation in which only those branches supplying the stomach are divided and the vagal nerve supply to the liver, gall-bladder, pancreas and small intestine is preserved. After a vagotomy, a drainage operation on the stomach is always carried out. This may be a *pyloroplasty* (Figure 41), in which the pylorus and the pyloric muscles are cut longitudinally and sewn up transversely, or a *gastrojejunostomy*, in which the antrum of the stomach is joined to the upper portion of the small intestine.

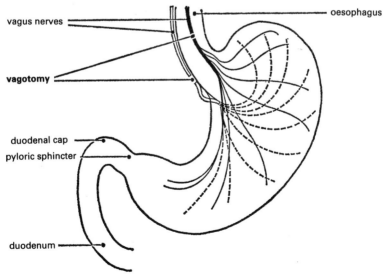

Figure 40 Truncal vagotomy

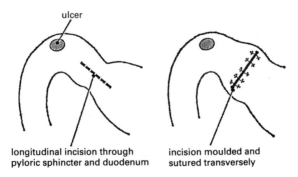

ulcer

longitudinal incision through
pyloric sphincter and duodenum

incision moulded and
sutured transversely

Figure 41 Pyloroplasty

The second way to reduce the acid output of the stomach is to remove the source of acid production, the parietal cells. This operation is called a *partial gastrectomy*. The more of the stomach that is removed, the greater will be the permanent reduction in acid production but, if too much is removed, the gastric reservoir may become too small, with serious consequences for the patient. The optimum amount of stomach to be removed is usually 60 to 70 per cent (Figure 42). Having done this, the surgeon closes off the duodenum completely. The first loop of intestine is then joined (*anastomosed*) to the cut end of the stomach, a procedure called *Polya* or *Billroth II gastrectomy* after two famous surgeons.

Polya gastrectomy
joining the stomach to the
jejunum

Billroth I gastrectomy
joining the stomach to the
duodenum

total gastrectomy
joining the oesophagus to
a Roux loop of jejunum
(stomach completely
removed)

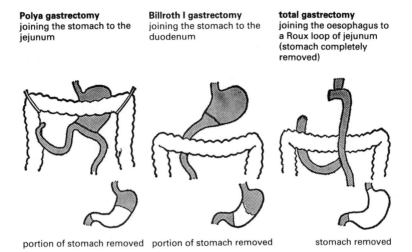

portion of stomach removed   portion of stomach removed   stomach removed

Figure 42 Various types of gastrectomy operation

Complications

The most urgent complication is *perforation*, which requires immediate operation to save the patient's life by stitching up (*suturing*) the perforation. This, of course, does nothing to cure the ulcer and further surgical treatment may be necessary at a later date. In many hospitals which specialize in the treatment of gastric disorders an emergency gastrectomy may be carried out for a perforated duodenal ulcer, if the patient's condition permits it.

Haemorrhage is discussed later under gastro-duodenal haemorrhage (see p. 74). *Pyloric stenosis* always demands surgical treatment, and this is undertaken after one or two weeks of intensive pre-operative preparation in hospital.

Pre-operative nursing care

The usual admission procedures are performed to give base-lines for medical and nursing intervention. Some patients will be severely dehydrated with consequent electrolyte imbalance. They may be anaemic and malnourished.

In such cases, these problems must be remedied prior to the planned surgery. Fluid can be replaced intravenously; if anaemia is severe a blood transfusion may be required, as this is the quickest way to restore haemoglobin although not without risk. If the patient is severely malnourished, a balanced intravenous diet may be given to restore the necessary calories, protein, vitamins and minerals that will be in deficit. Such an intravenous feeding protocol will be given via a central vein rather than a peripheral one, to ensure that the hypertonic fluids can be accommodated without interruption. If the nurse is unfamiliar with caring for a patient with a central venous line, she must seek advice and help to do this properly.

Occasionally, in cases of severe pyloric stenosis, the stomach should be washed out, as stagnant fluid will have been collecting there for some time, and it is potentially an infectious focus. In principle, there is no difference between stomach and rectal lavage, the latter being a more usual nursing procedure. A large-bore tube will be passed into the stomach via a nasogastric route (the tubes used for feeding are not sufficiently large to allow particles of food to be washed back so they would not be used). To assist drainage, the foot of the bed should be elevated and the patient made as comfortable as possible in that position – usually a left lateral position is most comfortable.

Initially, the gastric contents are aspirated, usually by a 50 ml syringe, and the total amount recorded as 'gastric residue' before lavage commences. Subsequently, an isotonic fluid – usually Normal Saline 0.9 % – is used for the lavage, but this may vary with the state of hydration and age of the patient. Washouts may be performed daily for a week or so, until the gastric return is clear.

This is an uncomfortable and distressing procedure for the patient. Much reassurance and encouragement should be given, with the reasons for its necessity.

Gastric ulcers

Gastric ulcers are quite different from duodenal ulcers. Small acute ulcers, the size of a pinhead, sometimes called *gastric erosions*, can occur in any part of the stomach in young people – usually as a result of taking too many aspirins or other similar drugs containing salicylates. They can cause severe epigastric pain and may even cause alarming haemorrhage. The other important cause is excessive alcohol intake. If the causative factor is removed, they heal up completely.

Chronic gastric ulcers may be benign or malignant. The *chronic benign ulcers* occur most commonly on the lesser curve of the stomach and in the *prepyloric* area. They occur in patients of a much older age group than do duodenal ulcers, and more often than not they are associated with chronic chest disease. If a gastric ulcer occurs on the greater curve of the stomach it will probably be malignant (probably 5 to 10 per cent of gastric ulcers which appear to be benign are in fact malignant).

The symptoms of gastric ulcer are similar to those of duodenal ulcer, but the patient always looks ill. The complications of gastric ulcer are perforation, haemorrhage and the liability to undergo malignant change. When these occur in a gastric ulcer they are far more serious than similar complications in a duodenal ulcer, usually because the patients are older, undernourished and often suffering from some other chronic illness.

Gastric ulcers are investigated in the same way as duodenal ulcers, but fibroscopy and biopsy are the most important procedures. Every gastric ulcer must be visualized directly and a biopsy of the ulcer taken.

Treatment

Once a gastric ulcer is diagnosed, it should be treated medically for three to four weeks. The healing of a gastric ulcer can be acceler-

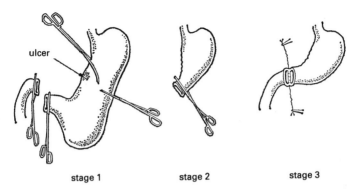

ulcer

stage 1   stage 2   stage 3

Figure 43 Billroth I gastrectomy. This example shows the treatment of an ulcer at a high level on the lesser curvature of the stomach

ated in only two ways. One is to give the drug *biogastrone* (an extract of liquorice) and the other is to abolish the smoking of tobacco. At the end of the course of medical treatment, a barium meal is given and fibroscopy is carried out to check that it has been successful. If the ulcer has not decreased in size, surgical treatment will be undertaken without delay. If a gastric ulcer recurs after healing, surgical treatment will also be needed. The reason for this is that, if a gastric ulcer recurs once, it will keep on recurring until it perforates, bleeds or becomes malignant. The aim of surgical treatment is to remove the ulcer, together with the antrum of the stomach. The gastric remnant is then anastomosed to the duodenum. This is called *Billroth I gastrectomy* (Figure 43).

Post-operative nursing care of duodenal and gastric ulcers

For the first 12 hours regular observation of vital signs should be monitored by the nurse. This gives early warning of internal haemorrhage. The nasogastric tube should be aspirated every hour, and the quantity and colour of the fluid recorded. Normally, the aspirate is stained with blood for the first 24 hours and then becomes clearer. Care must be taken with the intravenous infusion: accuracy in delivering the prescribed amounts and type of fluid and care to prevent infection of the site are essential.

When peristalsis returns to normal the nasogastric tube and intravenous infusion are removed, and gradually the patient can return to eating and drinking as usual. The passage of wind from the rectum indicates that the bowel is functioning normally again.

As with other surgery, details of specific instructions for individual patients cannot be included in a general text of this kind.

The nurse should read the doctor's instructions in the patient's notes regularly, and ask a senior member of the nursing staff or medical staff if she is still uninformed and therefore unable to carry out her care intelligently.

Gastro-duodenal haemorrhage

This is very important because it is quite common and because, especially in the elderly, it is a threat to life. The bleeding occurs when a peptic ulcer crater gets larger and exposes an artery running through the base. This artery becomes softened as a result of the associated infection and eventually erodes, with resulting haemorrhage into the stomach or duodenum. If the vessel is a small one, bleeding will be very slight and may not be noticed by the patient. The blood will be passed in the stools, but in such minute quantities that they remain of normal colour. But, if the stools are analysed in the laboratory and special tests are applied, blood (known as *occult blood*) will be found. The nurse may be asked to collect stools for this test and, if it is positive, it means that the patient is losing blood from the alimentary tract. Thus a person can become anaemic over a period of time. If the artery is larger, bleeding will be more severe and the patient will go to the doctor with a haematemesis (blood in the vomit) or melaena (blood from the bowels). In a young person, bleeding usually stops spontaneously because the artery retracts and closes the tear. In elderly people, however, the arteries are rigid and do not retract, so bleeding is likely to continue. Acute gastric ulcers (or gastric erosions) can cause severe haemorrhage, even in young people. Excessive intake of alcohol or drugs (such as aspirin) containing acetyl salicylic acid can cause these acute ulcers. Tumours of the stomach also bleed, sometimes for the same reasons as simple ulcers.

Symptoms

These all result from the loss of blood and include increasing weakness, pallor, thirst, a rapid thready pulse, cold clammy skin and falling blood pressure.

Treatment

Gastro-duodenal haemorrhage is an emergency. The immediate treatment is to restore the blood volume by blood transfusion. The nurse should keep an accurate 15 minute record of the pulse rate and blood pressure. These records, over a period of hours, will indicate whether the bleeding has stopped or is continuing. If bleeding has stopped, the patient is investigated and treated as for an uncomplicated ulcer. If bleeding continues despite adequate blood transfusion, emergency surgery will be necessary to save the patient's life.

Tumours of the stomach

The most common tumour of the stomach, and the most serious, is cancer (Figure 44). Benign tumours are rare, and cancer of the stomach is one of the most serious forms of cancer in the alimentary tract because there may be no symptoms whilst the growth is in a curable stage. Thus the disease is usually well advanced when the diagnosis is first made. One of the challenges to modern medicine is to try and diagnose this condition much earlier.

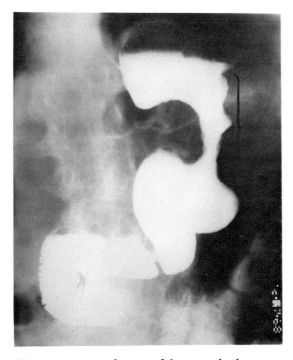

Figure 44 X-ray appearance of cancer of the stomach; the cancer causes a constant rigid deformity of the body of the stomach

Cancer can occur in any part of the stomach, and the symptoms it eventually produces will depend on the area of stomach affected. General symptoms such as weight loss, loss of appetite and increasing tiredness are late symptoms. If the growth is near the pylorus the symptoms will be those of pyloric stenosis (see p. 66). If the growth is near the cardia, difficulty in swallowing would be expected.

Some stomach tumours look like ulcers, some like cauliflowers, whilst others make the stomach wall very rigid and hard. Cancer of the stomach spreads to the lymph nodes which surround the stomach. It may spread to the liver, giving rise to secondary growths, and it may spread down the peritoneal cavity to the pelvis. When the patient is examined, there may be no physical signs or, on the other hand, the tumour may be felt in the epigastrium as a hard mass. An enlarged liver may be felt, which may sometimes be irregular due to the presence of secondary deposits. Barium meal and fibroscopy are the chief methods by which the diagnosis is made and the only form of treatment is surgery. The surgeon aims to remove that part of the stomach containing the tumour, together with a wide margin of normal stomach on either side. In addition, he must remove all the lymph nodes. The operation is called a *radical partial gastrectomy*. It is radical because not only is the cancer-bearing portion of the stomach removed, but also a good deal of the surrounding tissue to which cancer cells may have spread. This operation is much more extensive than partial gastrectomy for a simple ulcer. Sometimes the cancer is so huge and occupies such a large part of the stomach that the whole stomach must be removed; this is called *total gastrectomy*, which is a very

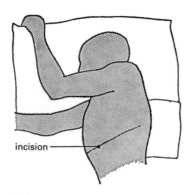

Figure 45 Position of patient and incision employed for total transthoracic gastrectomy

severe operation involving the opening-up of the chest as well as the abdomen (Figure 45). Following this operation a loop of small intestine is joined to the oesophagus (Figure 42) and, surprisingly, these patients can eat a perfectly normal meal when they recover.

If the growth is too far advanced when the surgeon opens the abdomen, much relief from vomiting can be obtained by the performance of a *gastro-enterostomy*. If occupied by tumour and the condition is completely inoperable, no surgical procedure is possible. However, a biopsy is always taken, firstly to confirm the diagnosis and secondly because in a very small percentage of cases the growth may be sensitive to radiotherapy.

Post-operative nursing care

Care is the same as that described for previous major surgery on the gastro-intestinal tract (see previous post-operative care). In the inoperable cases, beyond hope of surgical cure, the nurse meets one of her most severe challenges. It is important that she should not neglect these patients, but should do everything possible to comfort them and to relieve their pain.

Six
The peritoneum

Apart from the kidneys and pancreas, all the abdominal organs lie in the peritoneal cavity (Figure 46). The *peritoneum* is a continuous thin, shiny membrane which lines the abdominal cavity. It envelops most of the abdominal organs and forms the outer (*serous*) coat of organs such as the stomach and the intestines. The layer lining the abdominal wall is called the *parietal peritoneum*, and that covering the organs the *visceral peritoneum*. The outer or *parietal layer* of the peritoneum is richly supplied with nerves and is therefore very sensitive. The visceral layer, on the other hand, is poorly supplied with nerves and is insensitive. It has its own blood supply and can secrete serous fluid. The space between the parietal and visceral layers is called the *peritoneal cavity* and this cavity normally contains a fine film of serous fluid.

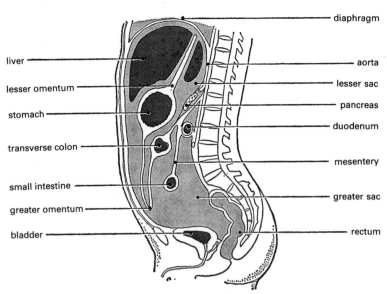

Figure 46 The peritoneal cavity

The most important portion of the peritoneum is the *great omentum*. This is a double fold of peritoneum which hangs down from the lower border of the stomach and loops up again to the transverse colon. It carries a great deal of fat and insulates the organs. It is sometimes referred to as 'the abdominal policeman', because it is frequently found adhering to inflamed organs. It seems to work its way towards them as though to prevent the spread of infection, in the same way that a blanket smothers a fire. Attaching the small intestine to the back wall of the abdomen is the *mesentery*. It is shaped rather like a fan – it has a very long border along which the bowel runs, yet it arises from a very short line at the back of the abdomen.

For descriptive purposes, the peritoneal cavity is divided into regions. The part above the transverse colon is called the *supracolic compartment* and contains the liver, stomach, gall bladder and spleen. The space between the diaphragm and liver is called the *subphrenic space* (pus can collect here to form a *subphrenic abscess*). The region below the transverse colon is referred to as the *infracolic compartment* and contains the complete small intestine and the pelvic organs. There are spaces in the pelvis between the bladder and uterus and between the uterus and rectum where, as a result of inflammation in the peritoneal cavity, pus can collect to form a pelvic abscess (see Figure 49).

The surface of the peritoneum is smooth and always kept moist with serum, so it prevents friction as the organs move against one another. The mesenteries of the peritoneum attach the abdominal organs to the abdominal wall. The transverse colon is attached by a mesentery called the *transverse mesocolon*. The peritoneum carries the blood vessels, lymphatics and nerves to the intestine, and these run between the two folds of the mesenteries. In disease the peritoneum acts as a warning and defensive mechanism for the gastrointestinal tract. Irritation of the parietal peritoneum, whatever its cause, will lead to abdominal pain for the peritoneum is richly endowed with nerve endings. Inflammation of any of the organs derived from the foregut (see p. 12) will cause pain referred to the upper abdomen or epigastrium. After several hours the pain may be generalized, but a knowledge of where it started will indicate which organ is at fault. Similarly, if any organ arising from the midgut is inflamed, the pain will first be felt around the umbilicus and will later be localized over the inflamed organ. A good example of this is acute appendicitis. The appendix is one of the organs derived from the midgut of the embryo. If it is inflamed, the onset of pain is around the umbilicus. A little later, the *parietal peritoneum* near the appendix becomes inflamed and the pain thus moves over to the right iliac fossa, the part of the abdomen lying directly over the appendix. Pain arising from the hindgut (the left half of the transverse colon, the descending colon, pelvic colon and rectum) is felt in the lower abdomen. Thus, pain arising from the peritoneum acts as a warning sign and the site of onset of the pain is the localizing symptom. Once inflammation starts in the peritoneal cavity, the peritoneum prevents it spreading. The greater omentum will wrap itself round the inflamed organ, and surrounding parts of the alimentary tract will adhere to it. If these measures fail, the peritoneum will pour out an enormous quantity of fluid in an endeavour to dilute the bacteria.

Peritonitis

This is an infection in the peritoneal cavity. The most common and most important cause is the escape of the gastro-intestinal contents into the peritoneal cavity. The gastro-intestinal tract contains millions of bacteria which are active in the digestive process; normally these make no contact with the peritoneal cavity, which is sterile. If, however, any part of the gastro-intestinal tract becomes diseased, its wall becomes infected and weakened. Should the wall rupture, the contents of the organ (containing virulent bacteria) will flood into the peritoneal cavity resulting in a *general peritonitis*. Perforated acute appentis is perhaps the most common

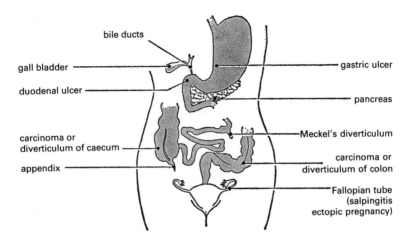

Figure 47 Sites of origin of diseases which may lead to peritonitis

cause of general peritonitis, but perforated gastric or duodenal ulcers are also common causes (Figure 47). A particularly serious one is perforation of the colon, as may occur in the condition called *perforated diverticulitis*.

Penetrating wounds (such as stab wounds) also cause peritonitis, for the injury leads to the escape of the gastro-intestinal contents. The urinary bladder may be ruptured by a direct blow such as a kick, especially if the bladder is distended with urine. Urine escapes into the peritoneal cavity and peritonitis is initiated. Similarly, if a patient has a large ovarian cyst and it ruptures, peritonitis will result. If the gall bladder is perforated by a stab wound, bile will escape into the peritoneal cavity. Bile is particularly irritant to the peritoneum and a virulent form of peritonitis results. The peritoneum pours out vast quantities of fluid to dilute the chemicals in the bile. As this fluid comes from the blood stream, the blood pressure falls dramatically. Patients in this condition are severely shocked, and treatment is extremely urgent if it is to be successful.

The escape of blood into the peritoneal cavity can also cause peritonitis since blood irritates the peritoneum. The most common example of this is a ruptured ectopic pregnancy (one in which an egg becomes implanted outside the womb and is then ejected). Another example is a tear in the mesentery carrying the blood vessels to the gastro-intestinal tract. In these cases, signs of internal haemorrhage will also be evident. A perforated duodenal ulcer is a good example of the way peritonitis can arise. The patient with this condition first experiences sudden, acute, severe and constant *epigastric pain*. This may be so severe that the patient collapses to the ground. This is the point at which the duodenal contents escape into the peritoneal cavity. If it is a large perforation and the stomach is full, the irritant fluid will quickly spread throughout the peritoneal cavity. The entire surface of the peritoneum will become inflamed and will respond in the usual way by pouring out an enormous quantity of fluid. Any movement of the patient will cause a worsening of the pain because of movement of the inflamed and sensitive peritoneum. The patient therefore lies quite still and his abdomen feels as hard as a board. This is because the muscles of the abdominal wall have contracted in an attempt to rest the peritoneal cavity and prevent undue movement. It is commonly described by doctors as 'board-like rigidity of the abdominal wall'.

At this stage, the infection in the peritoneal cavity may be overcome by the defence mechanisms of the peritoneum if the supply of toxic material from the perforation site is cut off. This can happen if the greater omentum plugs the hole in the duodenum, in which case it is known as the *first stage* of peritonitis. If the perforation is not sealed off, fluid will continue to pour out from the duodenum, overwhelming the normal response of inflammation. The *toxins* (poisons) flooding the peritoneal cavity will now be absorbed into the blood stream and all the intestine will be bathed in toxic fluid. The pulse rate and temperature will rise progressively, and the patient will look hot and flushed. This is the *second stage* of peritonitis. Because of the enormous fluid losses from the duodenum and the peritoneum, the patient will be dehydrated, he will complain of severe thirst, his tongue will be bone dry and his skin will be pinched. If nothing is done, the loops of intestine bathed in toxic fluid will become paralysed within 24 hours, losing all power of motility and becoming progressively more distended. The muscles of the abdominal wall are also affected by toxic absorption, and the previous muscle rigidity is superseded by a soft abdomen which becomes more and more distended. Because the intestines are paralysed they cannot propel their fluid contents onwards, which adds to the abdominal distension. The patient now begins to vomit as the fluid in the intestine is dammed back towards the stomach. This is the *third stage* of untreated peritonitis and is called *paralytic ileus*; the paralysed, distended, floppy intestine now contains several litres of stagnant fluid. The patient vomits copiously – repeatedly and effortlessly. He is too ill to move his head so that foul faecal-smelling fluid pours from his mouth. All the defence mechanisms of the body are now overwhelmed so that the pulse is imperceptible, the blood pressure is low and the temperature is well below normal. The patient becomes progressively more comatose and always dies. Even if treatment is vigorously started at this stage it will be unsuccessful because vital organs like the heart, kidneys and brain have been irreversibly damaged by the toxins now circulating round the body. Fortunately, this distressing condition is now rare because most patients seek medical advice at a very early stage of their illness.

In some cases, instead of contaminating the whole of the peritoneal cavity after perforation of an organ, the infection can be limited to the area around the perforated organ. This is known as *localized peritonitis* and happens when the defence mechanisms of the peritoneum seal off the perforation before the escaping fluid has had time to spread. This often occurs in small perforations of peptic ulcers, and in some cases of perforated appendicitis. The general condition of the patient remains good, and treatment is not required so urgently as in general peritonitis.

Symptoms and signs

The most important symptom of peritonitis is continual abdominal pain, but the signs which the patient displays vary according to the stage of the peritonitis. In the first stage, the signs of failure of the outposts of the circulation predominate – the skin is cold and pale, the pulse rate may be normal, the temperature may be normal or subnormal and the blood pressure is low. This state of affairs may last from one to several hours. In the second stage, the most important signs are the rapid deterioration of the patient's condition together with a rising temperature and pulse rate. Vomiting may occur. The third stage (*paralytic ileus*) occurs as described above.

Investigations

Peritonitis is easy to diagnose, although acute abdominal pain may not necessarily be due to peritonitis but rather to causes originating outside the abdominal cavity. If these cases are treated surgically, harm may be done. In some cases of pleurisy and pneumonia affecting the lower lobes of the lung, upper abdominal pain may be the only symptom and the upper abdominal muscles may be rigid. However, patients with pneumonia have a high respiration rate and usually have slight cyanosis (blue colour) of the lips and ears. Patients suffering from diabetes may complain of abdominal pain if their blood sugar is very high, and these cases can be distinguished from cases of peritonitis because diabetics have sugar in their urine.

Thus, the only investigations necessary in peritonitis are examination of the urine for sugar and a plain X-ray of the chest and abdomen (Figure 48).

Peritonitis can occur in patients who are being treated for a medical condition. This may be overlooked until a late stage, their abdominal pain being attributed to constipation or to something they ate. It is therefore important for the nurse to keep hourly pulse charts on all patients with abdominal pain, and remember that a rising pulse rate is always significant.

Treatment

All cases of general peritonitis invariably require an emergency operation for their relief. A number of essential measures must be carried out before an operation can be undertaken. The patient may have lost enormous quantities of fluid and be in acute circulatory

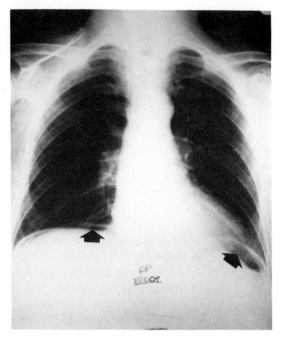

Figure 48 Erect X-ray of the abdomen showing free air beneath left and right domes of the diaphragm (arrowed)

failure. He will need intravenous fluid replacement urgently. Although several hours may have elapsed since the patient's last meal, the stomach may be full. A nasogastric tube should be passed, and the stomach contents aspirated. The nurse must note the quantity, colour and smell of the aspirate, and chart it carefully. Nothing must be given by mouth and the patient should be told why. Regular, refreshing mouth washes can be given, as although they will only have a local effect they will help to minimise the extremely unpleasant feeling of a dry mouth and, in a small measure, help to keep the mouth clean.

Analgesics should not be given for pain relief until the patient is seen by the doctor, as analgesics may mask the physical signs and delay the diagnosis. However, it may be necessary to report the patient's pain to the doctor on more than one occasion. If he is busy with other patients he may need reminding. It is unacceptable to leave a patient in pain for long. It may even enhance his symptoms if muscles are tensed.

Because of the acute abdominal symptoms and/or the dehydration, the patient may not be able to void urine in the normal way.

A urinary catheter may be required and, in view of the impending surgery, may be left in situ until the acute symptoms have subsided.

Localized peritonitis is not usually treated by emergency operation. The body has built a defence barrier around the inflamed or perforated organ and, in 90 per cent of cases, the inflammation will subside. To carry out an operation in these circumstances is to run the risk of converting a localized peritonitis into a generalized one. Furthermore, there is a considerable risk that the surrounding organs which are adhering to the inflamed site will be torn or damaged.

The principles of treatment are to rest the gastro-intestinal tract by complete bedrest and maintenance of nutrition via the intravenous route. Regular observations, dependent on the patient's condition, must be recorded. Similarly, observations of the patient himself should be made for signs of shock or pyrexia. If the patient is responding to the treatment, the pulse rate and temperature will return to normal and the abdominal pain will gradually decrease. Conversely, if the treatment is not succeeding, the abdominal pain will increase, the pulse rate will increase, the temperature will rise and the patient will vomit. These changes must be reported to the doctor at once, as they show that the infecting organisms are overcoming the body's defences, and surgery to allow drainage of the infected fluid may be necessary. Surgery to deal with the cause rather than the effect, may have to wait until much later, when the patient's general condition has stabilised.

Post-operative nursing care

Before undertaking the post-operative care of any patient who has had an emergency operation for general peritonitis, the nurse should as always read the surgeon's operation notes and take particular note of any special instructions. Emergency operations for general peritonitis are carried out in an area which is already infected, and infection in the wound is therefore common. The patient is afraid to move or to breathe deeply for the first few days, because of pain and this predisposes him to chest complications. Despite the most energetic suction during the operation and the presence of drainage tubes, some pus may still remain in the peritoneal cavity. This pus may form an abscess in the peritoneal spaces described above, particularly in the subphrenic space or in the pelvis (Figure 49). These *residual* abscesses may sometimes discharge spontaneously, but quite frequently need a second operation in order to drain them. If the infecting organism gets into the

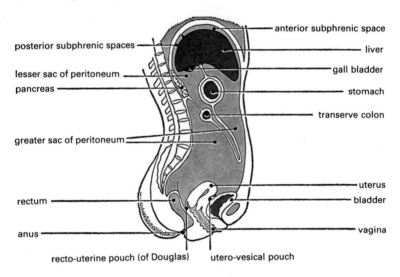

Figure 49 Sites of localized abscess formation complicating peritonitis

blood stream, septicaemia may develop. Following peritonitis, even in the immediate post-operative period, adhesions between loops of bowel can occur. These adhesions cause colicky pain and may obstruct the bowel.

The nurse is the first person to notice signs of recovery or relapse, and she should therefore monitor, check, observe and chart all vital signs and results of surgical intervention regularly and thoroughly. How regularly she does this will depend upon her experience in observing and caring for her patients. If she is unsure, she should check with someone more senior, as such decisions can only be made in the light of experience.

Specific attention should be paid to the intravenous infusion site, rate of drip flow and types of fluid to be infused. Observation of the wound and drainage tubes and of the patient himself are also important.

Seven
The liver, gall bladder and pancreas

THE LIVER

The liver, the chief storehouse and chemical factory of the body, is vital for life and is the body's largest gland. It is reddish-brown in colour and lies in the upper right quadrant of the abdomen just below the diaphragm. It has two lobes, a large right one and a smaller left one, each lobe containing millions of specialized cells (Figure 50). The liver has a rich blood supply. Pure arterial blood is brought by the *hepatic artery*, a large artery coming from the aorta via the coeliac axis. Inside the liver, this artery divides and subdivides to form a huge network of capillaries among the individual liver cells (Figure 51). In this way oxygen is brought to each cell to provide fuel for its work, and to sustain it. The liver has another supply of blood, that filled with the products of digestion from the gastro-intestinal tract and brought by the *portal vein* (Figure 52). This vein, which is very large, divides within the liver in a similar manner to the hepatic artery, so the products of digestion are brought to each liver cell (Figure 53). All the capillaries, both hepatic and portal, eventually drain into three veins called hepatic veins at the back of the liver. The hepatic veins drain into the inferior vena cava, which brings the blood back to the heart.

One of the many functions of the liver cells is to secrete a substance called *bile* into channels (*bile ducts*) which run between the liver cells. These bile ducts empty into *right* and *left hepatic ducts* which join just outside the liver to form the *common hepatic duct*. The bile formed in this way is stored in the *gall-bladder*; about two pints of this thick green fluid are secreted on average every day.

The liver is vitally concerned in the metabolism of the three principal food stuffs, carbohydrates, protein and fat (Figure 54). Carbohydrates reach the liver as glucose and fructose. If glucose is needed by the body, the liver will allow it to pass through. If it is

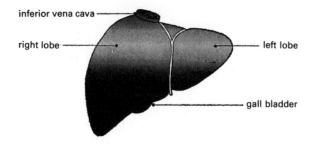

Figure 50 The general appearance of the liver

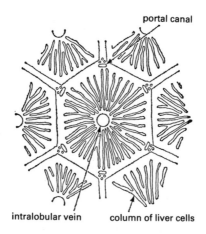

Figure 51 The minute structure of the liver, showing circulation

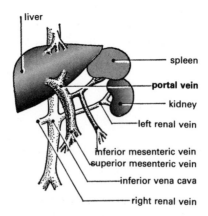

Figure 52 The normal anatomy of the portal vein

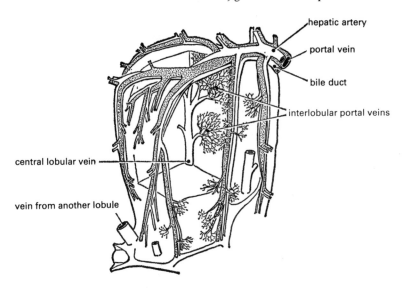

hepatic artery

portal vein

bile duct

interlobular portal veins

central lobular vein

vein from another lobule

Figure 53 Part of a liver lobule, showing the minute blood supply

not needed immediately, it will convert it and store it as the carbohydrate substance *glycogen*. There are always enormous stores of glycogen in the healthy liver, ready for any emergency. When it is needed, the glycogen is converted back to glucose in the liver and carried away in the blood stream. This function of the liver is controlled by a hormone called *insulin* secreted by the pancreas. If there is a lack of insulin in the blood, the glucose cannot be converted to glycogen, so too much sugar accumulates in the blood – this condition is called *diabetes mellitus*.

Proteins reach the liver in the form of their constituents, which are *amino acids*. These are the building bricks of the tissues of the body. Before passing them on in the blood stream, the liver rearranges these building bricks so that they conform to the individual pattern of a person's tissue. The wear and tear of the tissues must be continually made good, and this is effected through the liver. Any extra amino acids are mainly broken down by the liver to carbon dioxide and water. The nitrogen present in the excess amino acid is converted into a substance called *urea*, which is carried by the blood from the liver to the kidneys, whence it is excreted in the urine. If the kidneys are not functioning properly, the blood urea concentration will rise.

Fat reaches the liver in the form of fatty acids. The liver prepares the fat for combustion in the tissues by changing it chemically in a process called *desaturation*.

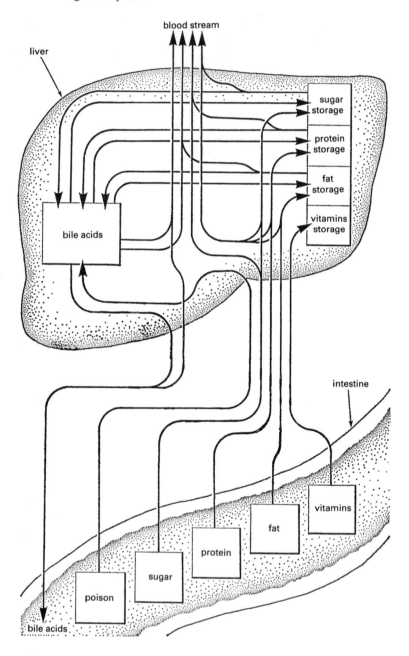

Figure 54 The movement of chemicals to and from the liver

Bile contains water, bile salts and bile pigments. The bile pigment is manufactured from worn out red blood corpuscles. Bile is a very important fluid, helping in the absorption of fats, and giving the colour to the faeces. Poisonous substances can be excreted from the liver via the bile. The liver also stores iron, the element which normally prevents anaemia, and it helps to break down worn out blood corpuscles. It plays a very important part in the defence mechanism of the body by producing *antibodies*. These protect the body against disease. The liver also manufactures the substance *heparin* which prevents clotting of the blood.

The liver is capable of achieving far more than is demanded of it. Three-quarters of the liver must be destroyed by disease before life is threatened and, if damaged, the liver has enormous powers of regeneration.

Liver disease

Symptoms

Mild inflammation of the liver results in a loss of appetite and a feeling of nausea. Patients suffering from this feel generally unwell and unduly fatigued. In mild cases this may be all but, in more severe inflammation of the liver, increasing drowsiness may occur and, in liver failure, the patient lapses into coma. In infection of the liver, shivering attacks (*rigors*) occur, and this is always serious. *Jaundice* (yellow dicolouration of the skin) is a frequent symptom of liver disease.

Injury to the liver

This usually occurs as a result of a crush injury to the upper abdomen or lower chest, for instance from a road traffic accident. Because the liver is soft, when it is crushed, multiple lacerations occur. A single laceration may result from a stab wound, and signs of internal haemorrhage will be present. The treatment is usually emergency operation and suture of the lacerations.

Inflammation of the liver

This is called *hepatitis*. The most important form, caused by a virus, is *viral hepatitis*. This may occur in a number of ways. Contact with a patient already suffering from the disease is common outside hospital, and epidemics may occur in this way. In hospital the virus may sometimes be transmitted from the blood of one person to another via syringes used frequently to take blood samples. If the syringes are inadequately sterilized, the virus may be transmitted in this way so, in most hospitals, disposable syringes are now used. Blood or plasma transfusions are also a hazard. Pooled plasma from many donors is frequently used. If any of the donors is suffering from even a mild form of viral hepatitis, the virus will be transmitted. Furthermore, the virus seems to gain in strength as it passes from person to person, and this explains why blood transfusion centres have such strict criteria in selecting donors. Every potential donor's blood is subjected to a rigorous series of tests before the donor is accepted. Hospitals in which heart and kidney transplants are carried out use enormous quantities of blood, and it is not surprising that outbreaks of viral hepatitis occur from time to time in these hospitals. The severity of the viral hepatitis varies considerably from the very mild to the fatal.

Treatment is always medical and the principle is to rest the liver and give plenty of carbohydrate and additional vitamin B by administering a diet of many small meals low in fat and rich in protein, and thus support the liver function whilst natural recovery takes place. Deepening jaundice and increasing drowsiness are danger signs.

Cirrhosis of the liver

This is a hardening of the liver. A cirrhotic liver is usually enlarged, very hard, tawny-brown in colour and the surface is covered with nodules (Figure 55). The most common cause of cirrhosis in Britain is *infective hepatitis*. In very severe attacks of infective hepatitis, the liver becomes swollen and inflamed and parts of it may die (become *necrosed*). The liver cells have extraordinary powers of repair and, if the patient recovers, extensive repair with fibrous tissue will take place. (This is like the scar tissue which forms after the skin has been cut.) The more extensive the initial liver inflammation, the more extensive the subsequent scarring, and the more likely the development of cirrhosis. The nodules on the surface of the liver represent the scarred areas. Similar changes take place in the liver if excessive amounts of alcohol are consumed over a long time, but excessive alcohol intake is often combined with a poor diet deficient in vitamins.

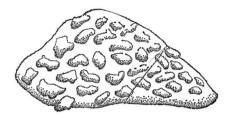

Figure 55 A cirrhotic liver; note the nodular appearance

If the cirrhosis is untreated, the normal liver cells will be replaced by more and more fibrous tissue. The liver will be unable to carry out its normal functions and a progressive state of chronic liver failure results. The patient becomes progressively more lethargic and jaundiced, and may lapse into *hepatic coma.*

At any stage of the disease the fibrous tissue may strangulate the veins running through the liver, forcing the blood back into the portal vein and its tributaries. This condition is called *portal hypertension* (Figure 56) and the portal venous blood, under high pressure, must seek an alternative route, bypassing the liver to reach the heart. There are many of these bypasses (*portosystemic anastomoses*) in the body, the most important being at the lower end

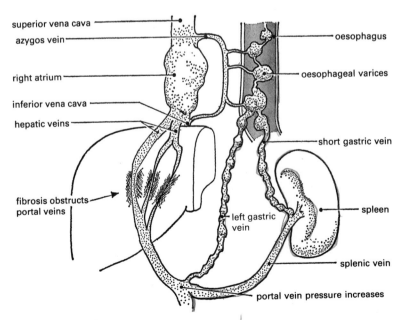

Figure 56 The cause of portal hypertension

of the oesophagus. In portal hypertension therefore, venous channels open up at this site so that blood at high pressure can escape into the systemic veins in the oesophagus, where the pressure is low. As more and more blood flows into these veins, they become distended and tortuous (like varicose veins in the legs) and are called *oesophageal varices* (see Figure 32). The chief complication of these veins is haemorrhage. The veins are very thin and bulge into the oesophagus. If they rupture, profuse haemorrhage will occur and the blood will be vomited up (*haematemesis*). Patients suffering from cirrhosis of the liver tolerate blood loss very poorly. The liver is already severely damaged, and the oxygen lack (*anoxia*) resulting from the blood loss may precipitate complete liver failure and death. It is because this complication of haemorrhage is potentially fatal that surgeons sometimes make artificial bypasses at less dangerous sites. The portal vein may be joined to the inferior vena cava where the two lie close together beneath the liver, an operation known as a *porta-caval shunt* or a portal-caval anastomosis (Figure 57). The portal blood at high pressure is shunted away from the dangerous area at the lower end of the oesophagus directly into the inferior vena cava, where it is safe. Other shunts may also be carried out but, of course, these only prevent further haemorrhage. They do nothing to lessen the natural course of cirrhosis.

Another effect of portal hypertension is that fluid can escape from the portal system of veins into the peritoneal cavity, causing a condition known as *ascites*. The high pressure in the veins over-

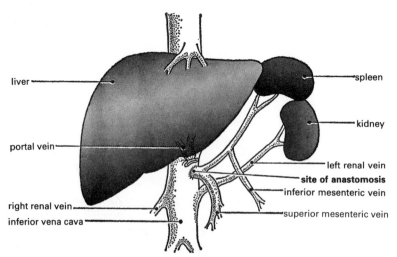

Figure 57 Porta-caval anastomosis; the portal vein is joined to the inferior vena cava

comes the osmotic pressure of the blood proteins, which normally holds the fluid back.

Liver failure can also occur suddenly or acutely. This is usually the result of overwhelming infection reaching the liver (e.g. when bacteria enter the portal system from any infected organ in the alimentary tract). In this way, neglected appendicitis may give rise to *portal pyaemia*. Multiple abscesses in the liver may also precipitate acute liver failure. In addition, certain drugs and anaesthetic agents can be poisonous to the liver. In the past, when chloroform was a common anaesthetic, acute liver failure occurred from time to time and, because of this, the use of chloroform has been largely abandoned. *Halothane*, a widely used modern anaesthetic agent, can be poisonous to the liver if employed on more than one occasion. Several other drugs are harmful to the liver, and it is wise to obtain from all patients admitted to hospital information about any drugs they are taking, especially if they are about to undergo an operation.

Treatment of liver failure

This depends on the cause of the liver failure and on whether it is acute or chronic. If it is caused by infection, antibiotic drugs offer the best prospects of cure. In chronic liver failure, dietary care and the use of drugs to lessen the formation of ascites are important. The nurse will supervise these treatments, keeping pulse and temperature charts and reporting any changes in the patient's general condition. If the liver fails, the kidneys will also fail because waste products, normally rendered harmless by the liver, accumulate. The amount of urine voided daily will gradually diminish in a patient with a deteriorating liver, and it will increase if the liver is recovering, so the nurse should ensure that the daily urine output is accurately recorded.

Cancer of the liver

Cancer can arise in the liver itself, but is extremely rare. However, secondary cancer in the liver from a primary growth in the alimentary tract is very common. This is not surprising, as blood from all the intra-abdominal organs is returned through the liver. Because cancer can spread via the blood stream, the presence of secondary cancer in the liver generally indicates a poor prognosis.

Tumours may be diagnosed during a *liver biopsy*, in which a small piece of tissue is removed from the liver for detailed examination (Figure 58).

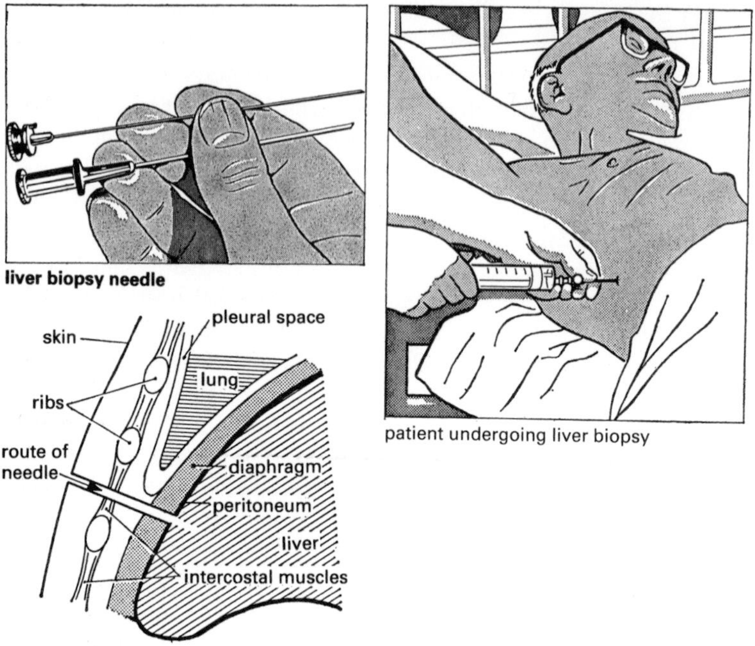

liver biopsy needle

patient undergoing liver biopsy

site, showing route of needle

Figure 58 Needle biopsy of the liver

Jaundice

This means a yellow discolouration of the skin. The explanation is quite logical. Bile is manufactured in the liver and excreted via the bile ducts into the duodenum. If there is an obstruction of any kind in the bile ducts, the bile is dammed back into the liver and will overflow into the blood stream. Bile contains bile pigments and these will be present in excess in the blood. In turn, these pigments will escape into all the tissues including the skin, giving it a yellow colour. This form of jaundice is called *obstructive jaundice*. If no bile pigments reach the intestine, the stools lose their characteristic brown colour and become clay-coloured. Some of the excess bile pigments circulating in the blood will be excreted in the urine, which will become very dark in colour.

The bile pigments are derived from worn out red blood corpuscles. The normal life of a red blood cell is about a hundred days. If these cells are broken down too quickly, the liver will not be able to cope with all the pigment it receives. Again, excessive bile pigments will overflow into the blood and jaundice will result. As it is caused by the too-rapid breaking up of the red cells (*haemolysis*), it is called *haemolytic jaundice*. This type of jaundice can affect newborn babies. There are other causes of excessive haemolysis of the red cells and these include snake bite and overactivity of the spleen. In the first case, the situation can be relieved with an antivenom serum, and in the second by removing the spleen.

The third form of jaundice is called *infective jaundice* and is caused by a virus infection in the liver which damages the liver cells.

The effect of jaundice is that the blood does not clot as quickly as it should. Vitamin K is essential for normal clotting, but this vitamin is not absorbed from the intestine in the absence of bile salts. Therefore, in obstructive jaundice, defective coagulation and haemorrhage can occur. This explains why jaundiced people bruise easily and why haemorrhage may be difficult to control during surgery. If the liver is severely damaged in the jaundiced patient, the urine output may fall. Skin irritation and itching are common complaints in jaundice and are due to excessive amounts of bile salts circulating through the skin. It will be found that jaundice causes depression and irritability, making the patients tearful and difficult to manage, but it should be remembered that this is part of the disease.

The level of jaundice can be assessed by measuring the amount of the pigment *bilirubin* in the blood. Normally this should not exceed 1 mg in every 100 ml of blood. In severe cases, it will be above 10 mg.

Pre-operative nursing care

Several days before the operation, vitamin K should be administered to lessen the risks of haemorrhage. As it is not absorbed from the intestine, the vitamin must be given by intramuscular injection. There is always some degree of liver damage in jaundice, and the nurse should maintain liver function by giving large quantities of glucose. This may have to be given by intravenous drip if the patient is nauseated. On the morning of the operation a solution called *mannitol* may be added to the intravenous drip. Mannitol is a *diuretic*, i.e. it increases the volume of urine secreted by the kidneys, and it thus protects the kidneys from failure during the operation.

Post-operative nursing care

The nurse's two most important duties following surgery are to watch for internal haemorrhage and to keep a very accurate record of the urinary output. A falling urine output is a most important warning sign, for it may mean that kidney failure has taken place. If the obstruction causing the jaundice has been relieved, then the stools and urine will gradually return to their normal colours.

THE GALL BLADDER AND BILE DUCTS

The gall bladder is a small pear-shaped bag, lying on the under-surface of the liver, which stores the bile secreted by the liver until it is needed. At any one time, the gall bladder could not possibly hold the two pints of bile produced daily, but this problem is solved by a unique property of the gall bladder. It can concentrate the bile at least twenty times. The mucous membrane of the gall bladder absorbs water from the bile, and this explains why the bile in the gall bladder looks very viscid. The gall bladder empties its bile into the common bile duct via a tube called the *cystic duct*. The cystic duct is provided with a two-way valve which controls the flow of bile into and out of the gall bladder. The cystic duct joins the common hepatic duct from the liver to form the *common bile duct* (Figure 59). This duct runs down behind the duodenum embedded in the head of the pancreas (Figure 60) and opens on the 'inner' wall of the descending limb of the duodenum. On the duodenum the opening is marked by a little mound (*papilla*) called the *ampulla of Vater*. The gall bladder obtains its blood supply from the hepatic

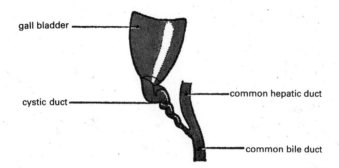

gall bladder

cystic duct

common hepatic duct

common bile duct

Figure 59 The gall bladder and bile ducts

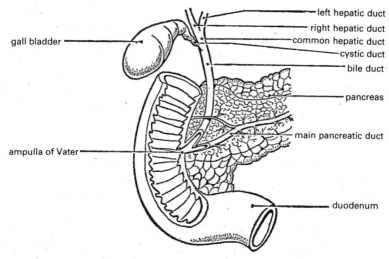

Figure 60 The relationship between the gall bladder, the duodenum and the pancreas

artery, and its blood drains into the portal vein, which connects with the liver.

Disorders of the gall bladder

Several diseases and disorders can impair the action of the gall bladder. Bacteria can gain entry either via the blood stream or by passing back up the common bile duct from the duodenum. This can result in inflammation, and is the most common lesion of the gall bladder. It may be either acute or chronic. Inflammation of the gall bladder frequently results in the formation of gall stones, especially if there is an obstruction in the bladder's outflow.

Gall stones

Gall stones form when there is an excess of cholesterol in the bile and there are insufficient bile salts to keep the cholesterol in solution. Bacteria present in the gall bladder may contribute by becoming the nucleus of the cholesterol gall stone. Gall stones are formed primarily in the gall bladder, but may migrate via the cystic duct into the common bile duct (Figure 61). Traditionally gall stones are more common in women, but they can occur in any patient, male or female.

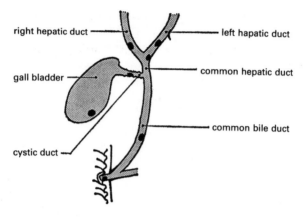

right hepatic duct — left hapatic duct

gall bladder — common hepatic duct

common bile duct

cystic duct —

Figure 61 The sites where gall stones may lodge

Symptoms

Pain is the chief symptom of gall stones. Because, in the embryo, the gall bladder developed from the foregut, the pain is located in the *epigastrium* (the region in the centre of the abdomen over the stomach, Figure 62), but it radiates to the right hypochondrium and may be referred to the tip of the right shoulder blade. It is colicky, comes on suddenly, and is usually aggravated by fatty food. This pain is called *biliary colic* and may be very severe, so severe in fact that the patient may writhe about the floor and vomit. Jaundice will only occur when a gall stone obstructs the common bile

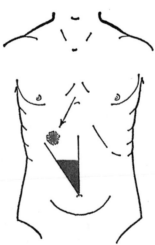

Figure 62 The pain felt in gall-bladder disease

duct. If acute inflammation (so-called *acute cholecystitis*) is present, the pain is constant and the patient's temperature is high. The abdomen will be tender and the muscles guarded in the upper right quadrant. Sometimes gall stones may become impacted, either in the neck of the gall bladder or in the cystic duct. In this case, the gall bladder will be unable to empty and will become progressively more distended as stagnant bile accumulates. This bile will inevitably become infected and produce a gall bladder full of pus. This is an *empyema* of the gall bladder, and the patient will suffer intense pain and have a high, swinging fever. If bacteria escape into the common bile duct, they may move up into the ducts of the liver, causing inflammation as they do so. This is *ascending cholangitis*. A patient with this condition will almost certainly be jaundiced, and rigors will occur.

In *chronic cholecystitis*, the symptoms and signs of illness are milder than in acute attacks. Patients complain only of indigestion, but it is usually found that they have vague pain in the upper abdomen, accompanied by bloating nausea and belching (*eructation*). These symptoms are aggravated by eating fatty food. In chronic inflammation of the gall bladder, these symptoms are so constant that they are named *biliary dyspepsia*. The gall bladder functions, but only poorly.

In about 1 per cent of patients who have had gall stones for a considerable time, cancer develops in the gall bladder; so, in rare cases, gall stones precede the development of cancer in the gall bladder.

Complications

The complications of gall stones are varied, but it is important to remember that they may be 'silent'. That is, some people harbour gall stones which only come to light during investigation of another complaint, and which do not produce any symptoms before they are discovered. However, gall stones tend to cause trouble sooner or later. As long as they stay in the gall bladder, acute or chronic cholecystitis may develop. Pus may form in the gall bladder, resulting in empyema. If a stone escapes into the common bile duct, biliary colic, jaundice or ascending cholangitis are all potential hazards. Repeated attacks of ascending infection can lead to changes in the liver, producing cirrhosis, so the liver becomes small and shrunken. If a gall stone becomes impacted at the lower end of the common bile duct, it may cause inflammation of the pancreas (*pancreatitis*, see p. 107). This is because the opening of the pancreatic duct lies very close to the ampulla of Vater and may easily become blocked.

If the gall bladder becomes very distended and blocked, the contents may be discharged into a neighbouring organ, such as the duodenum. First, it adheres to the duodenum. A gall stone will then burrow its way through both walls into the duodenum, creating an artificial opening (a *fistula*) between the two organs. The gall stone is then propelled onwards along the small intestine. When it reaches the narrowest portion of the small intestine, near the ileo-caecal valve, it may cause intestinal obstruction.

Investigation of gall-bladder disease

The doctor needs to find out whether the gall bladder is functioning, whether gall stones are present and whether any liver damage has occurred. A plain X-ray of the abdomen seldom reveals gall stones, for these only show up clearly on the X-ray if they contain calcium, which only about 5 per cent of them do. (On the other hand, 95 per cent of kidney stones contain calcium and are therefore easily visible on a plain X-ray.) To make it show up clearly, the gall bladder is outlined with a dye in an investigation called an *oral cholecystogram*. The patient is given a dye in tablet form on the evening before the examination. This dye is absorbed from the small intestine and is carried to the liver. The liver secretes it into the bile, from where it is concentrated in the gall bladder. If an X-ray of the gall bladder region is taken on the following morning, the gall bladder will show up, as it is full of dye (Figure 63). Its shape can then be examined and the doctor can determine whether any filling defects caused by gall stones are present. The gall bladder functions by concentrating the dye. The patient is now given a fatty meal to see if the gall bladder contracts as it should in response to fat. A further X-ray is taken half an hour later to see whether this has happened. If the gall bladder is diseased, it fails to concentrate the dye. However, this investigation is of little value if the patient is jaundiced since, in this case, the liver will not take up the dye. The nurse must ensure that the dye is actually taken in the correct amount at the right time. If the patient vomits the tablets, then the ward sister or doctor must be informed.

The state of the bile ducts are investigated by an *intravenous cholangiogram*. In this investigation the patient is given the dye in the X-ray department by intravenous injection. X-rays will then be taken at frequent intervals.

Liver function is investigated by carrying out a series of liver

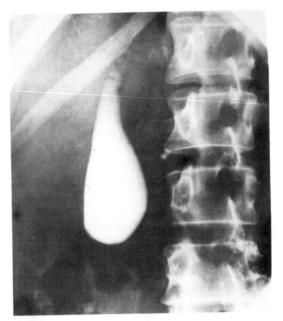

normal

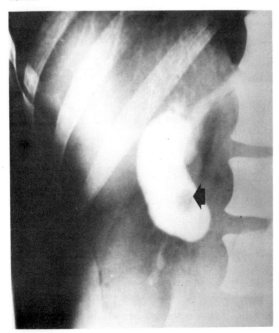

gall stone

Figure 63 Cholecystograms; the gall bladder is outlined with the dye

function tests. These are biochemical tests on blood samples, which are analysed in the laboratory. A piece of liver tissue can be obtained for examination under the microscope without operation. This is called needle biopsy of the liver (see Figure 58), and is carried out in the ward. Because the liver has such a rich blood supply, the nurse's most important duty is this investigation is to watch out for signs of internal haemorrhage when the procedure has been completed.

Treatment

Bed rest is the normal treatment for *acute cholecystitis*. *Pethedine* is administered to relieve the pain and antibiotics to overcome the infection. Fluids only are given by mouth. In this way, most cases settle down. If investigations show that gall stones are present, the gall bladder can be removed weeks later when all inflammation has subsided. Occasionally, however, an emergency operation is needed – e.g. if empyema of the gall bladder develops. In this case simple drainage of the gall bladder (*cholecystostomy*) is carried out (Figure 64). The most serious complication of acute cholecystitis is ruptured of the gall bladder resulting in biliary peritonitis, and the nurse should be constantly aware of this possibility.

When gall stones are diagnosed, especially when they are giving rise to symptoms, they will always be removed, together with the gall bladder. If the gall bladder were left behind, further stones would re-form. Removing the gall bladder removes the stones, the sources of the stones and a potential site for a new growth. The operation for the removal of the gall bladder is a common one and called *cholecystectomy*.

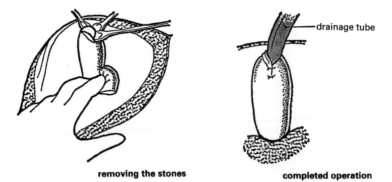

removing the stones   completed operation

Figure 64 Cholecystostomy.

Pre-operative nursing care

This is the same as described previously, for major abdominal surgery. The usual problem of convincing the patient that deep breathing will help prevent chest complications, and not cause disruption of the surgical scar etc., are highlighted in this operation. This is due to the proximity of the gall-bladder to the underside of the diaphragm, and therefore thoracic cavity (see Figure 63).

The cholecystectomy operation

Before the gall bladder is removed, the surgeon ensures that the bile ducts do not contain any stones. The bile ducts are therefore X-rayed during the operation (an *operative cholangiogram*). A catheter is passed into the common bile duct via the cystic duct, and a dye is injected which shows up any gall stones which may be present. To remove these stones, the common bile duct is opened. Following removal of the gall bladder, a corrugated rubber drain is always let down to the liver bed to drain away any oozing of blood or bile that may occur. If the bile duct is explored, it will be drained by a T-tube which drains bile into the receptacle by the patient's bed. The short limbs of the T-tube are placed in the bile duct, and the long limb is brought out through the skin.

Post-operative nursing care

In addition to the normal pulse, blood pressure and temperature charts, the nurse must take special care with the drain following cholecystectomy. The T-tube may be removed by the surgeon or one of his colleagues, but it is usually removed by the nurse. In principle, it is no different from removing any other kind of drainage-tube, but considerable traction may be needed to retrieve it because of its T-shape. The nurse should not be afraid to pull hard and firmly. To proceed gingerly will usually cause more distress to the patient; it will take longer, and may not be successful. If a T-tube is present, it is normally left in position for ten days. During this time, bile will drain continually into the drainage bag by the bed. The amount should be measured and recorded daily. If drainage ceases, the tube has either come out of the bile duct or has become blocked. This complication should be reported immediately. Before the tube is removed on the tenth day a further X-ray (a *T-tube cholangiogram*) is taken to ensure that the lower end of the common bile duct is patent, with full flow into the duodenum. The T-tube may now be safely removed since, if bile dose trickle out for a day or two, it will do so via the fibrous track formed by the tube and not into the peritoneal cavity. As for other abdominal operations. fluids and diet are resumed gradually, as the individual patient's condition allows.

THE PANCREAS

The pancreas is a gland with two functions. It produces a hormone called *insulin,* which is secreted into the blood stream, and an external secretion called *pancreatic juice* which passes down the pancreatic duct and empties into the duodenum along with the common bile duct. The pancreas looks rather like a flask lying on its side, and is situated across the upper abdomen behind the stomach (Figure 65). The rounded end is in the curve of the duodenum and the tip extends across almost to the spleen. The pancreatic juice is produced by numerous small lobes (*saccules*) of the gland, and collects into a main duct which runs the length of the pancreas.

The pancreatic juice plays an important part in the digestion of foodstuffs in the small intestine through the action of its enzymes *trypsin, amylase* and *lipase*. Insulin is produced by groups of cells

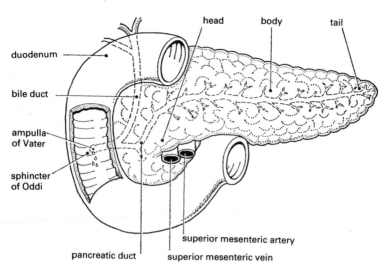

Figure 65 The pancreas

lying between the saccules of the gland, which are richly supplied with blood capillaries and are called *islets of Langerhans*.

Insulin is essential to life and controls the metabolism of carbohydrates by enabling the liver to store glucose. If there is a deficiency of insulin, a condition known as *diabetes mellitus* results. If the liver cannot store glucose, there is an excess of this substance in the blood which runs to waste in the urine. In this situation, the body has to use fat as fuel instead of glucose. But fat cannot be burned completedly without glucose, and the result is that *acetone bodies* are made which are composed of incompletely burned fat. Acetones bodies are poisonous and, when they are formed, the diabetic will sink into a coma unless insulin is given.

In recent years another hormone, indistinguishable from gastrin (the hormone of the stomach), has been isolated from cells in the pancreas. If these cells grow too large, an enormous oversecretion of gastric acid will be produced from the stomach.

Disorders of the pancreas

Acute pancreatitis

This is a most interesting and potential dangerous disease and usually results from blockage of the main pancreatic duct. When this occurs, the pancreatic secretions are dammed up behind the obstruction until the saccules within the gland rupture, releasing the potent enzymes trypsin, lipase and amylase, which can respectively digest proteins, fats and starches. When the enzymes escape from the pancreas into the surrounding tissues, they digest them. In Britain, the most common cause of obstruction is a gall stone impacted in the ampulla of Vater. The patient complains of a sudden onset of upper abdominal pain, usually after a heavy meal, and vomits copiously. The pain radiates around to the back (the pancreas lies behind the peritoneum). The pulse and temperature are raised and the abdomen is very tender to the touch, but not rigid as in a perforated peptic ulcer. Cases of acute pancreatitis are thus normally admitted to hospital as 'acute abdomen' cases. It can be difficult to distinguish pancreatitis from general peritonitis, and a period of observation is very valuable. During this period of observation, there are two tests which can be very helpful. The amount of the enzyme amylase in the blood can be measured – in acute pancreatitis this is usually higher than normal. The level of the enzyme diastase in the urine can also be measured and it, too, is usually elevated. If the diagnosis is certain, acute pancreatitis is best treated by medical means. An operation is carried out only if the patient continues to deteriorate despite adequate medical measures. The principles of medical management are to rest the pancreas, to diminish the pancreatic secretions, to relieve pain and to give an antibiotic to overcome any secondary infection.

The nurse must make sure that the patient takes nothing by mouth. If the stomach and duodenum remain empty, there is no stimulus for the pancreas to secrete. To ensure this, a nasogastric tube must be passed and aspirated continually. The pancreatic secretion can be further diminished by giving large doses of the drug *atropine*, which inhibits the secretion. Pain is relieved by giving pethedine. An antibiotic sensitive to a wide range of bacteria will be prescribed.

If surgery is performed, only simple drainage is carried out. The most important factor in the post-operative care of these patients is to protect the skin from the digestive and destructive power of the pancreatic enzymes.

Chronic pancreatitis

This may follow repeated attacks of acute pancreatitis. The pancreas is largely replaced by fibrous tissue, with the result that the volume of pancreatic juice is much reduced. If the head of the pancreas is involved in chronic pancreatitis, jaundice may occur from strangulation of the lower end of the common bile duct by fibrous tissue. If the secretion of the enzyme *lipase* is diminished, fat will not be digested properly and will appear in the stools giving them a pale, greasy appearance. This is called *steatorrhoea*. These patients are sometimes in a good deal of pain which is difficult to relieve. Treatment of the condition is also difficult. Sometimes, if the disease is confined to the head of the gland, the obstructed portion can be short-circuited by linking the gall bladder to the duodenum. In this way the jaundice is relieved and the lack of pancreatic enzymes can be made good in the diet.

Cancer of the pancreas

Cancer of the pancreas occurs most commonly in the head of the gland. This is a most serious form of cancer, for two reasons. Firstly, the only symptom it produces is painless jaundice. Although the only symptom, it is a late symptom and does not appear until the growth has completely surrounded the common

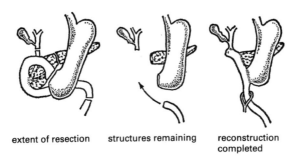

extent of resection   structures remaining   reconstruction
completed

Figure 66 Pancreatectomy

bile duct. Secondly, once the growth gets outside the capsule of the
pancreas, it invades vital blood vessels (such as the portal vein and
the hepatic artery) nearby, which makes it incurable by any form
of surgery. The symptoms are, quite simply, those of obstructive
jaundice. In the few fortunate patients who can be operated on at
an early stage of the disease, the head of the pancreas can be
removed. The remainder of the pancreas is implanted into the small
intestine, and the operation is called *pancreatectomy* or *pancreatico-
duodenectomy* because the duodenum must also be removed (Figure
66). If the growth cannot be removed by this major operation, jaundice can be relieved by allowing the bile to reach the intestine by
an alternative route. The gall bladder can be thus anastamosed to
the duodenum or to a loop of small intestine. These are called
palliative operations.

Eight

The small intestine

The small intestine is concerned with the digestion and absorption of food. Its structure, particularly that of the mucous membrane and the two muscle layers (see Figure 2), is perfectly adapted to these needs. The small intestine starts at the pyloric sphincter, which opens into the duodenum. This is horseshoe-shaped, is about thirty centimetres long and receives the opening of the common bile and pancreatic ducts. The duodenum ends behind the stomach, where the jejunum begins. The jejunum which is altogether two and a half metres long, lies coiled in the peritoneal cavity attached to the posterior abdominal wall by its mesentery. It continues as the ileum, which is about four metres long. This is also coiled (Figure 67) and it ends at the ileocaecal valve situated in the right iliac fossa. The small intestine secretes the intestinal juice (the *succus entericus*), containing water, salts and enzymes. Any germs absorbed from the small intestine are collected and destroyed by collections of lymphoid tissue lying just below the mucous

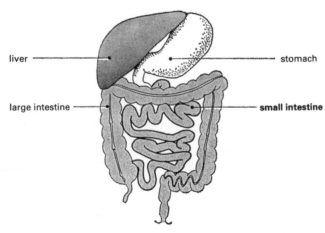

Figure 67 The small intestine

membrane. These collections of lymphoid tissue in the ileum are called *Peyer's patches* and, in typhoid fever, they become inflamed.

The mucous membrane of the small intestine

The liquid contents of the gut must be brought into very close contact with the mucous membrane, so the membrane must have an extremely large surface area. To achieve this, the mucous membrane is thrown into folds (*valvulae conniventes*) which run round the circumference of the bowel. If, throughout the small intestine, all these folds were straightened out, the lining would be approximately thirty metres long. The mucous membrane is covered with hair-like *villi* for the absorption of food into the blood stream. The mucous membrane also contains the intestinal glands, which secrete the intestinal juice.

The blood supply to the small intestine is derived from one major artery, the *superior mesenteric artery*, and arises from the front of the aorta. This is a very important artery. In the embryo, it is the original artery of the midgut and therefore supplies all those structures which are developed from this. The artery supplies the whole intestine through a system of branches which form arcades of vessels in the mesentery and subdivide into a capillary network beneath the mucous membrane. The intestine has only one source of blood supply and, if the artery is blocked at its origin, the whole intestine will be deprived of blood and die. But, if the blockage occurs lower down, the result will not be so serious. This is because there is a large overlap of arterial supply amongst the mesenteric arcades. The venous blood drains into the veins which accompany the arteries, and these eventually unite to form the *superior mesenteric vein*, which drains into the portal vein.

The total volume of intestinal juice secreted every day is three litres. In the normal intestine, most of this is reabsorbed into the blood stream lower down in the intestine (in the colon) and therefore dehydration does not occur.

Congenital disorders

During development, the alimentary tract first forms as a simple tube. This tube then divides into three parts. The stomach and first part of the duodenum develop from the front part of the tube (the foregut). The small intestine develops from the central portion (the midgut). The midgut is straight at first, but it grows very rapidly, so rapidly that the foetal abdominal cavity is soon too small for it, and the midgut extrudes itself outside the cavity and continues to grow thus. In the embryo, the midgut communicates with the part of the alimentary tract inside the abdomen via a tube called the *vitelline duct*. Later, the midgut returns to the abdominal cavity and accommodates itself by coiling up. It remains in this position up to the adult stage. This explains why some parts of the intestine lie in front of others.

In the embryo the tube is not hollow, but is packed with cells. As it grows, small gaps appear between the cells and these gradually coalesce to form the lumen of the intestine.

The development of the small intestine is a complex process, and occasionally, something may go wrong. Parts of the tube may remain solid or fail to canalize. This is known as *atresia* of the intestine and will show up in the newborn baby as intestinal obstruction. Sometimes part of the intestine may duplicate itself; in other words, two channels may be formed instead of one. This is known as *re-duplication of the gut*. When the developing intestine returns to the abdominal cavity, the coiling or rotation may not be complete. Thus, on rare occasions, the appendix may be found on the left side of the abdomen instead of in its normal, right-hand position, a situation known as *malrotation of the gut*. Normally the vitelline duct shrivels up and disappears before birth but, in about 2 per cent of people, part of it persists as a connection (*diverticulum*) in the terminal ileum. It is called a *Meckel's diverticulum* and is about five centimetres long, resembling the appendix. Like the appendix it may become inflamed, and the symptoms and signs are similar to those of appendicitis.

Obstruction of the small intestine

The most common and most urgent surgical condition which occurs in the small intestine is obstruction. It is always more severe than obstruction of the large intestine because of the enormous amount of fluid lost through vomiting. The obstruction may be *complete*, causing an acute condition, or *incomplete*, causing a chronic form of obstruction. There are only three basic reasons why obstruction should occur in the small intestine:

(a) The lumen may be completely blocked. This may come about if a foreign body is swallowed, or because of a gall stone. The blockage usually occurs at the narrowest part, which is the ileum.

(b) The wall of the tube may be altered by disease. In some diseases, such as Crohn's disease, the wall of the intestine becomes thickened, narrowing the lumen. Tuberculosis may be followed by a localized stricture which would also narrow the lumen. Another cause may be *intussusception*; here, a length of the intestinal tube is telescoped into the next section and is drawn further and further in by the action of the intestinal muscles (Figure 68). This is not uncommon in the first year of life.

(c) Pressure may be exerted from outside the intestine, causing obstruction. Examples of this are an obstructed hernia or the twisting of a loop of intestine so that its contents are obstructed; the latter is known as *volvulus* (Figure 69).

Whatever the cause, the signs and symptoms of acute small-bowel obstruction are typical. The patient first complains of abdominal pain. All pain originating in the small intestine is referred to the periumbilical region, and the pain is felt there. It

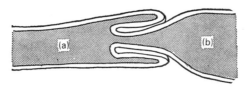

Figure 68 Intussusception. Section (b) has invaginated itself into section (a)

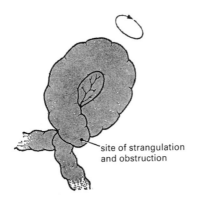

Figure 69 Internal strangulation (volvulus of the small intestine)

is a colicky pain which varies in intensity, rising to a crescendo and then fading away, but repeatedly recurring. Vomiting then occurs, and it is significant if it is progressive. In progressive vomiting, the stomach contents are first returned, later the vomit is bile-stained and later still it is foul-smelling fluid from the part of the small intestine above the obstruction. This brown fluid is sometimes (incorrectly) known as faecal vomit. It is stagnant and smells like faeces but, in fact, is not faeces and is more properly called *faeculent* or faeces-like vomit.

Absolute constipation is usually found in acute small-bowel obstruction, i.e. no air or faeces are passed after the administration of two enemata. Two are given because faeces below the obstruction may be passed after the first enema.

The abdomen is not usually distended, except in the very late cases of obstruction. If the abdominal wall is thin, *peristalsis* (movement of the intestine) may be observed. The outline of the loops of the small intestine can be seen contracting vigorously in an attempt to propel the intestinal contents past the obstructed area. If an obstructed hernia is the cause of the blockage, a tender irreducible swelling can be seen and felt at one of the hernial orifices.

An even more serious and urgent form of small-bowel obstruction is *strangulating obstruction*, in which the blood supply to the obstructed part is cut off. If this is not rapidly relieved, the bowel will become gangrenous and death will follow. This type of obstruction is associated with continuous pain and abdominal tenderness.

If the intestinal obstruction is not treated, the end result is exactly the same as with untreated generalized peritonitis, namely paralytic ileus. The progressively distending bowel will become paralysed and a vicious circle will become established.

Investigations

The doctor usually makes a correct diagnosis by investigating the history and examining the patient. A plain X-ray of the abdomen is taken to confirm that the small intestine is distended (Figure 70). In this, multiple fluid levels in the distended bowel can be seen. If the patient has been vomiting a good deal, signs of dehydration and even acute circulatory failure may be evident. The degree of dehydration should be assessed as soon as possible after the patient has been admitted to the ward. Examination of the urine will show that it is very concentrated and has a high specific gravity. This is because the kidneys preserve as much water as possible, to counteract the fluid lost through vomiting. Blood samples are taken to

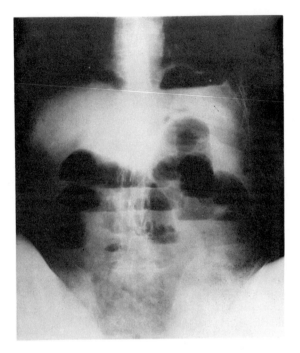

Figure 70 X-ray appearance of the abdomen in obstruction of the small intestine, showing multiple fluid levels in the dilated loops

estimate the serum electrolytes and urea. This investigation shows which salts have been lost by vomiting and stagnation in the obstructed loops of bowel, and determines the type of fluid to be replaced by intravenous drip.

Treatment

Intestinal obstruction carries a high mortality rate, particularly in the elderly, and an emergency operation is usually needed to relieve the obstruction. However, the eventual success will depend on careful preparation of the patient before the operation and good post-operative nursing care.

Pre-operative nursing care

After the patient has been admitted to the ward, an intravenous drip should be set up, and a nasogastric tube is passed. The intravenous drip is used to replace the water and salts lost by vomiting and thus correct the dehydration and also the electrolyte imbalance. If there is time, this should be corrected before the operation. The nasogastric tube is very important. This is because the stomach is always full of fluid in intestinal obstruction – hence the vomiting. Under an anaesthetic, this fluid may well up into the oesophagus and spill over into the trachea causing an aspiration pneumonia which would almost certainly be fatal. The nasogastric tube, carefully passed into the stomach, is used to aspirate this fluid before the operation. The amount, colour and odour of the fluid obtained should be entered on the fluid balance chart. It may be necessary to aspirate at fifteen-minute intervals, as intestinal fluid will regurgitate back into the stomach until the obstruction is relieved. Many difficulties in passing the nasogastric tube can be avoided if the patient understands why the tube is being passed and is allowed to swallow it gently. It should never be forced down his throat.

If the patient is in severe pain and the diagnosis has been established, the drugs *pethidine* or *omnopon* may be given intramuscularly. If the doctor has not seen the patient and reached his diagnosis, no painkilling drugs (*analgesics*) should be given, as they may mask the signs and delay the diagnosis. The patient's blood pressure will be low on his arrival in the ward, but this will be restored to normal when the circulatory failure has been corrected.

The operation

In the operating theatre, the simplest procedure necessary to relieve the obstruction is carried out. This may entail merely the division of a band or obstructing adhesion. If, however, the small intestine is gangrenous, the operation becomes much more serious. The gangrenous portion must be excised and an end-to-end anastomosis made between the healthy ends of the intestine. If the obstruction is caused by irremovable malignant disease, it may be relieved by carrying out a short-circuit operation. A side-to-side anastomosis is made between healthy intestine above and below the obstruction. If there is marked abdominal distension, the surgeon may have difficulty in closing the abdomen.

Post-operative nursing care

The general care of the patient following surgery for small-bowel obstruction is similar to that after any abdominal operation. If the obstruction has been successfully relieved, the volume of aspirate from the nasogastric tube will gradually decrease and become clearer. However, this may not happen immediately because, although the obstruction has been relieved, the bowel wall may have developed a temporary paralysis as a result of the distension. The real sign of a successful operation is the passage of wind (flatus) from the rectum. This indicates that the intestine has begun to work normally again. It is essential that the nurse maintains an accurate fluid balance chart and adheres to specific, prescribed fluid intake instructions, as outlined in the introductory nursing chapter. The importance of this cannot be over-stressed. As before, the nasogastric tube will remain *in situ* until normal intestinal function has returned.

Inflammatory diseases

Gastro-enteritis

This is the most common acute inflammatory disease of the small intestine. It can occur at any age, but it is especially dangerous in infants because of the high mortality rate.

The lining of the stomach and intestine becomes swollen, reddened and inflamed, and pours out enormous quantities of fluid. The patient complains of crampy pain in the centre of the abdomen, vomiting and profuse diarrhoea. If this is not treated, rapid dehydration will follow. The disease is extremely serious in infants because they cannot tolerate rapid loss of fluid from the body.

In Britain, drinking infected milk or some other fluid is the most common cause of gastro-enteritis. Outbreaks tend to occur in hot weather if ordinary hygienic standards break down. Newborn infants have not had time to build up their defence mechanisms against the bacteria that cause enteritis, so it is vitally important to sterilize the feeding bottles when nursing these babies. Other causes of gastro-enteritis are dysentery, cholera and typhoid fever. These are caused by specific microorganisms. Typhoid fever causes ulceration in the lower part of the small intestine, and these ulcers occasionally perforate, leading to peritonitis.

Nursing care

The diagnosis of gastro-enteritis is made by examining a specimen of stool in the laboratory. The nurse should collect a specimen of stool and ensure that it arrives in the laboratory in a fresh condition and not dried up, otherwise the pathologist will not be able to identify the organisms. An accurate fluid balance chart should be kept, and the quantity and quality of each stool recorded. An antibiotic is usually prescribed, and must be given at the exact time and route indicated. Otherwise, insufficient blood-levels of the drug will result, and there will be a poor therapeutic effect.

In those cases who do not respond to oral medication, intra-venous antibiotics will be prescribed.

The nursing of infective patients needs special care to prevent the infection spreading from one patient to another. This is known as *barrier nursing*. The infection can spread by direct contact, by communal use of utensils, by failure to sterilize the hands before treating the next patient, and in many other ways. In many cases, this scrupulous care needs to be carried out in special hospitals devoted entirely to infectious diseases.

Staphylococcal enteritis

Another important form of enteritis is staphylococcal enterocolitis. This has appeared since the introduction of antibiotics and can occur post-operatively in any patient who has had large doses of antibiotics before the operation. It is caused by flooding of the alimentary tract by staphylococci which are resistant to penicillin. The patient develops fever and severe diarrhoea, and rapidly passes into a cholera-like state of dehydration. This requires massive intra-venous infusion but, even with energetic treatment, the mortality is high. So, if any patient develops diarrhoea following an operation on the gastro-intestinal tract, it should be reported immediately.

Crohn's disease

Crohn's disease is an inflammatory condition of the wall of the terminal ileum, also known as *regional enteritis*. The cause is unknown and the treatment depends on the symptoms it produces. The disease causes a thickening of the bowel wall and is found in two main forms. One is an *acute* condition, in which both the bowel wall and the mesentery are swollen with fluid (*oedematous*) and the affected area looks red and thickened. The second is the *chronic* form, in which a tubular stricture has formed and there is hyper-trophy and dilation of the bowel proximal to it. The affected bowel may stick to other coils of the small intestine, the transverse colon and the bladder, and an abnormal communication (*fistula*) can occur between these adherent organs (Figure 71). The mucous mem-

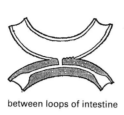
between loops of intestine

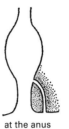
at the anus

Figure 71 Fistula formation in Crohn's disease

brane, seen under the microscope, has a typically cobblestoned appearance.

Symptoms

The acute form of Crohn's disease is like acute appendicitis occurring over weeks and months instead of hours or days. The chief symptoms are central abdominal pain, fever, loss of appetite, nausea, loss of weight and looseness of the bowels. In the chronic form, loss of weight and attacks of subacute intestinal obstruction occur.

Special investigations

A special X-ray examination called a *barium follow-through examination* is usually carried out (Figure 72). This examination is necessary because Crohn's disease tends to affect multiple segments of the small intestine, and areas of normal bowel (known as *skip areas*) occur between the diseased segments.

Treatment

In the absence of a known cause, most cases of Crohn's disease are treated medically. But, if medical treatment fails to control the disease or if complications occur, surgery will become necessary. Complete bed rest is essential in the acute phase. A patient suffering from Crohn's disease always looks ill and toxic. The temperature and pulse rate are raised and abdominal discomfort adds to the misery. The most encouraging sign that the patient is responding to treatment is a progressive fall in the temperature and pulse rate. A variety of drugs may be used to reduce the inflammation in the small bowel.

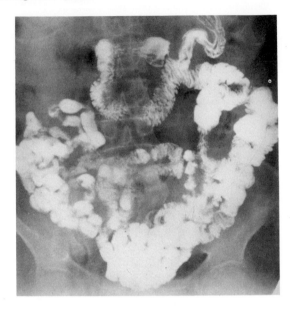

normal mucosal pattern

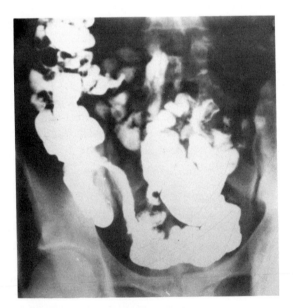

stricture in the ileum due to Crohn's disease

Figure 72 X-ray of barium follow-through

The drug *salazopyrine* has a non-specific anti-inflammatory effect and *cortisone* acts by inhibiting the formation of fibrous tissue. The antibiotic *ampicillin* combats secondary infection, and *codeine phosphate* will reduce the number of stools passed. Patients are often anaemic, and blood transfusion may be necessary. The diet should be rich in calories and vitamins. It is possible to give a 2000–3000 calorie diet in liquid form, using a liquidizer. Vitamins A, B and C can be added and help to promote healing in the tissues. The team, consisting of doctors, nurses, a dietician or nurse-nutritionist, is essential in the nutritional management of these patients.

Nursing care

The long periods of bed rest may be irksome to patients with Crohn's disease, as these are often young people, many of them young mothers concerned about their children. The nurse should help them understand why bed rest in essential.

A stool chart should be kept, recording the number of stools passed daily, their colour and consistency. The nurse should discover if the patient is free from pain or suffers attacks of colic. If the patient is having *cortisone* therapy, the pulse rate should be watched carefully. Cortisone masks peritonitis but, if the pulse rate rises, this may indicate peritonitis and should be reported immediately. Encouraging signs are weight gain (the patient should be weighed weekly), falling pulse rate, falling temperature and decrease in the number of stools.

Complications of Crohn's disease are intestinal obstruction, fistula formation and perianal soreness, so the anal region should be examined daily and any redness or swelling reported. If urinary symptoms develop, a fistula may have formed between the small bowel and the bladder.

Surgical treatment

Crohn's disease is frequently discovered during an operation for a condition diagnosed as acute appendicitis. If this happens, a biopsy is taken and the abdomen is closed without further surgery. Medical treatment is then started. In the chronic form of the disease, the affected segment of bowel may need to be removed or resected and continuity is restored by joining the ends of the bowel together. This may involve a very large resection if multiple segments of bowel are involved. If there are multiple fistulae and

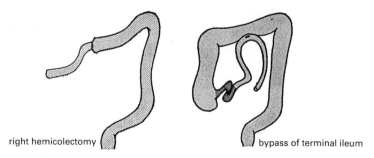

right hemicolectomy   bypass of terminal ileum

Figure 73 The main types of operation for Crohn's disease of the ileum

dense adhesions, resection may be very dangerous, so the diseased segments are short-circuited, allowing them to rest and heal more readily (Figure 73).

Post-operative nursing care

This is similar to the post-operative care of small-bowel obstruction. But patients with Crohn's disease are more likely to develop complications, as they are chronically ill; the intestine may take a long time to regain its motility, and the intravenous drip and naso-gastric suction may need to be continued for longer than usual. Accurate fluid balance charts must be kept. If the patient was being treated with steroids before the operation, the wound will need particular observation for signs of wound infection, since steroids delay healing.

Tuberculosis of the small intestine

This is usually secondary to open tuberculosis of the lung. Tuber-culosis of the small intestine arises because of the tubercle bacillus gains entry to the intestine via the stomach when sputum is swal-lowed. The microorganisms may cause ulcers in the wall of the ileum. Unlike other ulcers, tuberculous ulcers are usually multiple and are situated crosswise in the bowel. When these ulcers heal they cause strictures in the ileum.

Symptoms and signs

The patient with tuberculosis of the small intestine may be known to have active tuberculosis of the lung and experience attacks of intermittent abdominal pain with diarrhoea. These may be accom-panied by loss of weight and fever. If a stricture occurs, the symptoms will be the same as those of intestinal obstruction with colicky abdominal pain and vomiting. The patient will almost certainly be admitted to a surgical ward.

Special investigations

Every patient admitted to hospital with an acute condition should have a chest X-ray taken. This will reveal tuberculosis of the lung, even if the patient's past history is not known. If this disease is active, there may well be associated abdominal symptoms. Samples of the sputum should be taken for examination for the presence of tubercle bacilli. The bacilli may also be discovered by the examination of gastric washings. These should be obtained first thing in the morning before the patient has had anything to eat or drink. This is because the patient swallows a good deal of sputum during the night, and this will be present in the stomach in the morning.

If there is no obstruction, the patient may be given a barium meal for a barium follow-through examination of the small intestine. This may reveal a stricture or an ulcer.

Treatment

Cases of active tuberculosis of the lung are best treated in specially equipped hospitals. Treatment consists of bed rest, a nutritious diet and the use of anti-tuberculous drugs. These patients may have to spend a long time in hospital, and the nurse should help them to overcome the boredom.

If intestinal obstruction is present, surgery may be necessary to short-circuit the affected bowel. The pre- and post-operation care is the same as in cases of intestinal obstruction.

After the operation, the treatment of tuberculosis with drugs continues. The nurse must ensure that these are given at the correct times and in the correct amounts. The rehabilitation of the patient will start before he leaves hospital and will involve the assistance of the hospital social worker.

Summary of the operations on the small intestine

Enterectomy

A loop of small intestine is removed, and the two ends sewn together again. The operation is carried out for a gangrenous small bowel or following injury. It is also carried out for some cases of Crohn's disease and tuberculosis. Important points of post-operative care are the hourly aspiration of the stomach to relieve any distension above the anastomosis, and adequate intravenous fluid replacement until the bowel regains its motility.

Entero-anastomosis

One portion of the small intestine is short-circuited into another portion beyond a diseased section or pathological lesion without removing the lesion. This is a less severe operation than enterectomy. The two portions of bowel are simply sewn (*sutured*) together side by side, to exclude the diseased portion. The common indications for this operation are an irremovable obstruction, such as severe adhesions not causing gangrene, and those cases of Crohn's disease and tuberculosis unsuitable for resection. The post-operative nursing care is the same as that following an enterectomy.

Feeding jejunostomy

A feeding jejunostomy is carried out if, for any reason, it is anticipated that the patient will not be able to eat normally for some time or if feeding by mouth is impossible because of an injury to the oesophagus. A small incision is made in the upper abdomen, a loop of the upper jejunum is found and a very small opening is made in it. A balloon catheter is inserted through this hole and sutured in position. The other end of the catheter is led out through the abdominal wall (Figure 74). After the operation, nothing at all should be introduced into the catheter for the first 24 hours. A fluid diet should be ordered to make up 3000 calories per 24 hours from the diet kitchen. Twenty-four hours after operation, a little glucose

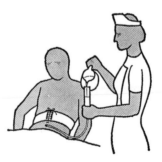

Figure 74 A patient receiving food through a jejunostomy

and water may be introduced into the catheter at hourly intervals. On the third day, the fluid diet can be given at hourly intervals.

At first a little food should be given often. If too much is given at any one time, the patient will experience severe nausea, complain of feeling faint and weak, and diarrhoea will almost certainly occur. These are symptoms of dumping. If this occurs, the feed should be halved. In time, the feeds will be tolerated quite well. The patients should be taught to feed himself through his feeding jejunostomy tube, as he will be the best judge of how much fluid he can tolerate at any one feed.

Nine
The colon and rectum

The large intestine runs from the ileocaecal valve to the anus. The part beyond the ileocaecal valve is the *colon*, which ends at the beginning of the rectum. It is described in five parts – the *caecum*, the *ascending colon*, the *transverse colon*, the *descending colon* and the *sigmoid colon* (Figure 75).

The *caecum* is the blind end of the colon lying in the right iliac fossa. It is shaped like a pouch, and the ileum enters it from the side. The opening is guarded by the ileocaecal valve. The appendix is attached to the caecum at its base. It is often a site of inflammation because its wall contains a good deal of lymphoid tissue.

The *ascending colon* runs up from the caecum on the right side to the undersurface of the liver, where it turns to the right (in a bend called the *hepatic flexure*) to become the *transverse colon*. This loops across the front of the abdomen below the stomach until it reaches the spleen, where it forms the *splenic flexure*. From this, the *descending colon* runs down on the left side of the abdomen to the left iliac fossa. Here the colon forms an S-shaped bend known as the *sigmoid colon*. This runs into the pelvic cavity and leads into the *rectum*. The rectum pursues a tortuous course through the pelvis

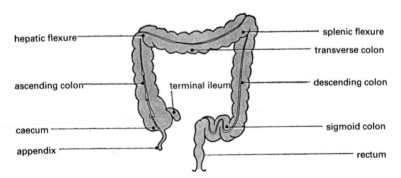

hepatic flexure

ascending colon

terminal ileum

caecum

appendix

splenic flexure

transverse colon

descending colon

sigmoid colon

rectum

Figure 75 The colon, seen from the front

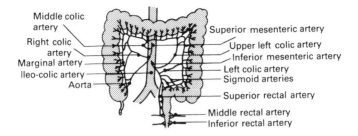

Middle colic artery
Right colic artery
Marginal artery
Ileo-colic artery
Aorta

Superior mesenteric artery
Upper left colic artery
Inferior mesenteric artery
Left colic artery
Sigmoid arteries
Superior rectal artery
Middle rectal artery
Inferior rectal artery

Figure 76 The arteries supplying the colon and rectum

and changes direction three times. The spurs formed at each turning point are called the *valves of Houston*. When the rectum is visually examined with an instrument known as a *sigmoidoscope* (see Figure 77), these spurs must be carefully negotiated with the instrument.

Like the small intestine, the wall of the colon consists of four layers. However, in the colon, the longitudinal muscle layer is gathered into three bands instead of forming a complete coat. These three bands are called *tacniae*; they draw in the wall where they lie, and it pouches out between them giving the colon a characteristic puckered appearance from the outside.

The blood supply of the right side of the colon comes from the superior mesenteric artery via branches arising from its right-hand side. The most important of these branches are the right colic and mid colic arteries (Figure 76). The reason for this is that, in the embryo, the right colon develops from the midgut and must therefore be supplied by the artery of the midgut. On the other hand, the left colon develops from the hindgut, whose artery is the inferior mesenteric. This artery supplies all the left colon and the sigmoid colon by branches called the left colic and sigmoid arteries. The arteries of the left and right colon are connected with each other through small vessels running around the margin. Surgeons rely on these marginal arteries to maintain the blood supply when one or other of the major branches leading to the colon has to be tied off.

Functions of the colon

The colon has two functions. It transports waste material from the alimentary canal out of the body and, during this process, absorbs water from the waste material (*faeces*). This not only helps to conserve the body's water, but also gives the stools a suitable consistency for evacuation. Normally, the faeces are pushed along the colon by peristaltic waves, a slow process. However, if the ileum suddenly empties its contents into the caecum, the whole colon contracts and faeces are forced through the sigmoid colon into the rectum. This normally happens following the intake of food into the stomach and is called the *gastro-colic reflex*. When the rectum bcomes distended with faeces, the desire to defaecate is experienced. The passage of faeces through the colon is accelerated when the activity of the muscles is increased. This occurs when the mucous membrane is inflamed, as occurs during infection by dysentery and in ulcerative colitis. The passage of faeces through the colon is an automatic process until they reach the rectum. The desire to defaecate is a reflex act, but it can be inhibited voluntarily and then the desire passes away. This commonly occurs if it is not convenient to empty the bowel when the reflex occurs. If, however, the desire to defaecate is repeatedly neglected, the nerve impulses from the distended rectum no longer initiate the defaecation reflex. The colon dilates and becomes very floppy, and the rectum and lower colon become filled with hard faeces. Evacuation may occur only at intervals of weeks, and it will require enemata and increasing amounts of purgatives to empty the rectum and colon. Elderly people, confined to bed for long periods, may neglect the desire to defaecate for so long that large, hard concretions of faeces may become impacted in the rectum. This may cause a partial obstruction in the large bowel. Many such cases of *faecal impaction* are to be found in geriatric wards. Above the obstructing mass of faeces, the colon cannot absorb water. Liquid will therefore escape around the impaction, and the patient will complain of diarrhoea. This paradox is called *spurious diarrhoea*.

The colon and rectum in disease

The two functions of the colon may be interrupted by disease. Passage of faeces may be interrupted by spasm or so-called *organic stenosis* of the colon. At first, the bowel muscle above an obstruction contracts more powerfully. The muscles of the colon are less powerful than those of the small bowel, so the colon is less effective in the face of obstruction; it dilates more readily and the pain is less. The caecum is the first part to dilate and can become enormously distended. Distension of the abdomen is thus much greater in large-bowel obstruction than in small-bowel obstruction.

Any inflammation of the lining (*mucosa*) of the bowel decreases water absorption. As well as this, the lining produces an excessive amount of mucus. If the inflammation is generalized, diarrhoea will result.

Symptoms and signs of large-bowel disease

The symptoms of large-bowel disease vary with its position. If the caecum is obstructed, for instance, the symptoms will be similar to those of a lesion in the terminal ileum. Colicky abdominal pain is therefore common in this case because there is not so much colon to dilate and accommodate the small-bowel contents. Nausea and vomiting occur, and weight loss and general ill health are common. On the other hand, lesions in the distal colon rarely give rise to digestive upsets and the patients do not feel unwell. A most significant symptom in colon disease is a change in the bowel habit. Obstruction is intermittent in the early stages, so recurring constipation, becoming progressively more severe, is common. If the obstruction is in the right colon, there will be enough normal mucosa beyond the obstruction to absorb water from the fluid faeces when the obstruction is temporarily alleviated. Diarrhoea is therefore not a regular symptom in obstruction of the right colon. On the other hand, when an obstruction in the pelvic colon is temporarily overcome, large quantities of fluid faeces are released into the short segment of colon beyond. This segment is unable to absorb all the water, and this accounts for the alternating bouts of constipation and diarrhoea typical of lower-colon obstruction lesions.

While generalized inflammatory diseases of the colon give rise to diarrhoea, localized areas of inflammation (depending on the site of the inflammation) need not necessarily do so. Inflammation in the caecum may not give rise to any change in the bowel habit, whereas inflammation in the pelvic colon (as in *diverticulitis*) may give rise to diarrhoea because the rectum is unable to absorb all the water and mucus discharged from the inflamed pelvic colon.

Some of the symptoms of colon disease can be explained by the nature of the lesions causing them. Cancers of the colon are usually infected and exude varying quantities of mucus, serous fluid and pus. This exudate will be absorbed by the rest of the colon in cancers of the proximal bowel, and the stools may be normal. But, in cancers of the rectum, this portion of the bowel constantly fills with exudate, and this triggers off the defaecation reflex. The patient complains of passing small, frequent, loose, slimy stools. He constantly attempts to empty his bowel, but is unable to rid himself of the desire to defaecate. This symptom, which is usually painful, is called *tenesmus*.

Cancers and inflammatory lesions of the colon bleed easily. *Rectal haemorrhage* is thus a common symptom in patients with tumours or inflammatory disorders of the colon and rectum. The bleeding can present itself in several ways. In cancer of the caecum, the blood is so intimately mixed with the faeces that it is not noticed by the patient. However, the blood loss may cause a severe anaemia, and symptoms of this may therefore be the ones brought to the doctor's attention in this form of cancer of the bowel. Bleeding from a cancer of the pelvic colon will coat the stool with blood, and so will be easily noticed. The doctor needs to determine the colour of the blood lost. Blood from a cancer high in the colon will be partially changed by the stool and will be dark in colour, whereas the blood from a cancer low in the pelvic colon or rectum will be bright red in colour.

Investigations in large-bowel disease

The investigation of the colon and rectum, like all other investigations, starts with a thorough investigation of the patient's history and a physical examination. Particular attention is paid to symptoms such as a change in the bowel habit, diarrhoea, the passage of blood, mucus, pus or slime. A digital examination of the rectum is always carried out by the doctor and will give detailed information about the last ten centimetres of the rectum, as well as information about the pelvic organs. Any abnormal stool should be saved by the nurse for the doctor's inspection, as useful information can often be obtained from it. *Special investigations* include *sigmoidoscopy* and types of *barium enema*.

Sigmoidoscopy

The sigmoidoscope is a long hollow tube measuring thirty centimetres in length (Figure 77). The upper rectum, rectosigmoid junction and lower pelvic colon can be visualized directly through the sigmoidoscope, and this is always used when investigating large-bowel disease. No preparation of any kind is necessary for diagnostic sigmoidoscopy, and no enema or suppository needs to be given beforehand. In sigmoidoscopy (Figure 78), the doctor is looking for evidence (such as an excess of mucus, the presence of blood, ulceration or neoplasm) of disease in the mucosa. If an

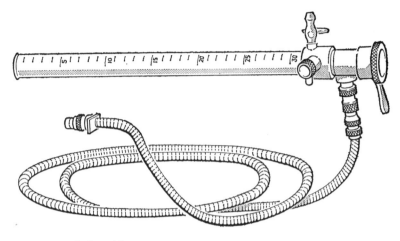

Figure 77 A sigmoidoscope

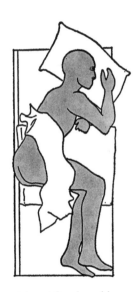

Figure 78 The patient positioned for sigmoidoscopy. The left hip rests on a small sandbag and the buttocks project slightly beyond the edge of the table

enema or suppository is given beforehand, this evidence may be washed away, and the resultant liquid stools will obscure the view. Abnormal-looking areas in the mucous membrane of the rectum should always be biopsied with a biopsy forceps (Figure 19). If the patient understands beforehand what is involved, he will relax during the sigmaidoscopy. However, in many patients the recto-

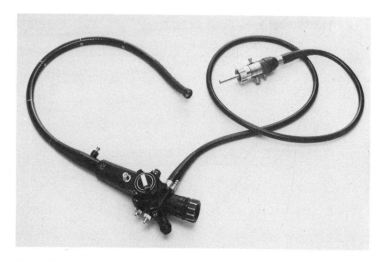

Figure 79 A flexible fiberoptic sigmoidoscope

sigmoid junction is too sharply angulated to allow the rigid instrument to be passed. The advent of the modern fiberoptic flexible sigmoidoscope (Figure 79) has overcome this problem and is better tolerated by the patient. With this instrument, however, all faeces must be removed prior to examination otherwise the lens will be soiled by faecal material and views will be obscured. A colonoscope (Figure 80) is a longer version of the flexible sigmoidoscope and enables all areas of the colon, in many cases as far as the caecum, to be inspected and biopsied.

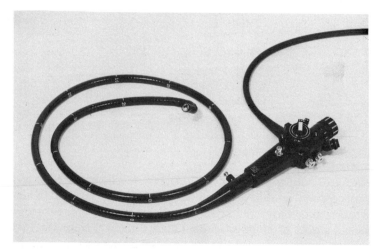

Figure 80 A flexible fiberoptic colonoscope

Barium enema

If barium – which is radio-opaque – is injected into the large bowel as an enema, the anatomy of the colon can be seen on an X-ray and most abnormalities detected (Figure 81). The radiologist observes the colon on the X-ray screen as the enema is injected. This examination is very useful for the right and left sides of the colon, but is of little value for lesions in the rectosigmoid region, as the pelvic colon overlaps this area. However, this area is always within reach of the sigmoidoscope. Sigmoidoscopy should always be carried out before the barium enema is arranged.

A *double-contrast enema* is a refinement of the ordinary barium enema. If air is injected into the colon partially filled with barium, a double-relief picture is obtained. The lumen of the bowel appears black, and small tumours – otherwise invisible – project into it as a white outline because they are coated with barium.

Preparation for a barium enema is important in order to obtain an empty colon, and aperients should be given for two nights before the examination. When the patient arrives in the X-ray department, a colonic washout is given before the barium is injected. This washout should be as thorough as possible to avoid having to repeat the operation because detail was obscured by residual faeces.

Colostomy

A great many conditions of the colon require an operation to open the large bowel and drain its contents out of the body. This is known as a *colostomy* and, because it is used to treat so many conditions, it is described in detail here before the diseases themselves are described.

A colostomy may be necessary in order to prevent the faecal stream from reaching a segment of the colon where it may do harm, for example, following wounds of the colon or rectum, to prevent leakage of faeces or as a preliminary measure in resection of the colon in order to allow the join to heal. Faeces may have to be diverted away from an inflamed portion of the colon (as happens in *diverticulitis* to allow the inflammation to subside. The second important reason for performing a colostomy is to provide an exit for the faeces when the normal route is not available. Examples of such a situation are in acute obstruction of the colon (where the operation prevents rupture of the bowel) and after complete removal of the rectum.

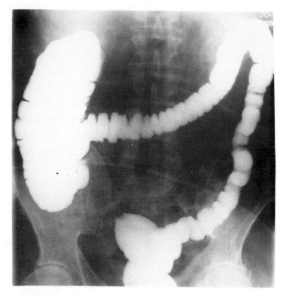

a normal colon

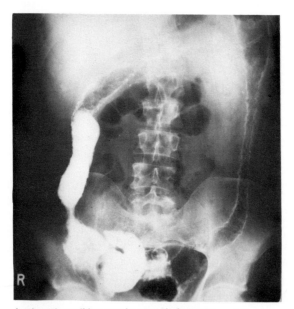

in ulcerative colitis: note the smooth, featureless colon

Figure 81 X-rays of barium enemas

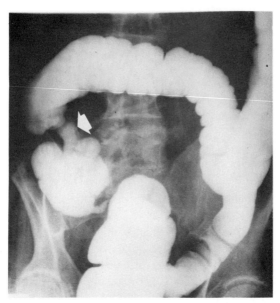

showing a typical filling defect in carcinoma of the colon,

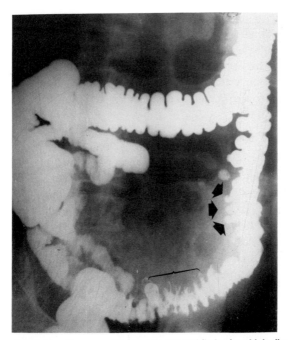

diverticular disease: note both separate and (below) multiple diverticula

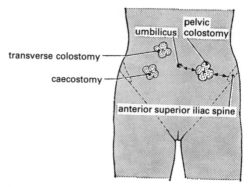

Figure 82 Colostomy sites

There are two main types of colostomy, a *loop colostomy* and an *end colostomy*. These may be temporary or permanent.

A *loop colostomy* is made by bringing a loop of mobile colon through the abdominal wall. A glass rod is placed beneath the loop to prevent it from retracting back into the peritoneal cavity. A loop colostomy can be made in the mobile parts of the colon, namely the transverse and pelvic colons. When a loop colostomy is opened, there are two openings. The faecal stream will emerge from the upper (proximal) opening. The distal opening is inactive.

An *end colostomy* is usually made in the left iliac fossa, following resection of the rectum. The lower descending colon is brought out through the abdominal wall and sutured to the skin (Figure 82). There is only one opening (*stoma*) in an end colostomy.

Pre-operative nursing care

Patients will understandably be very concerned about having a colostomy, and will need time to accept the idea, and longer to accept the effect it will have on them and their lives. If permanent, such changes in body image can have a profoundly demoralising effect, and occasionally, an individual will deny the obvious presence of the colostomy, and never accept it.

However, in time, and with the help of a patient and understanding nurse, the majority of patients cope very well, and return to near normal function.

The nurse can do much to allay anxiety and teach the patient new coping strategies. She must move at the patient's pace, however, and not suggest to him how he should feel and be reacting. The patient feels what he says he feels.

Preparation of the colon and rectum for surgery

The safety of colon and rectum surgery depends on preparation. The problem of operating on the colon is that it has a much poorer blood supply than the small intestine. If a join is made between two parts of the colon, healing is slower and the risk of leakage is far higher. The aim of colon preparation before surgery is to minimize these risks.

Normally, the vast numbers of bacteria in the bowel cause no harm but, if they escape into the peritoneal cavity, they behave in a most virulent manner. The main organism in question is the bacillus *E. coli*. This is not sensitive to penicillin, but can be inhibited by the sulphonamide drugs. In preparing the patient for surgery, the number of organisms in the colon can be significantly decreased by giving an insoluble sulphonamide such as phthalysulphathiazole (*thalazole*) by mouth for five days. This drug is not absorbed from the colon, so it acts locally. It takes five days to sterilize the bowel, giving the thalazole in divided doses of 2 g every six hours, and this is the reason patients are admitted to hospital five days before the operation.

During this pre-operative period, the colon and rectum should be emptied of all faeces by giving colon washouts. A colon washout is quite different from an enema, and involves giving four and a half litres of warm water via a long rectal tube so that the water reaches the splenic flexure. Sometimes the faeces are so hard that colon washouts alone are not sufficent, and laxatives or aperients are also given by mouth. All this time, the patient should be given a low-residue diet and, for the last 48 hours, fluids only are allowed.

If there is an obstructing lesion in the colon, it will not be possible to empty the faeces above the obstruction, so the surgeon will almost certainly need to carry out a preliminary colostomy. The colon is prepared in the way described above, and the colon above the obstruction is washed out via the colostomy and below it via the rectum. In addition to giving thalazole by mouth, a liquid form of the drug must be instilled through the distal limb of the colostomy. The definitive operation is then carried out as a second stage.

Post-operative nursing care

Colostomies are opened on the operating table. When the patient returns to the ward, a disposable plastic bag is in position. During the first 24 hours, there are three very important observations to be made. The first is to note whether excessive bleeding is taking place from the colostomy edge. Secondly, the colour of the mucosa must be examined. It will be pink if the blood supply is adequate. If the mucosa becomes progressively darker or even black, it will eventually slough off. Lastly, a check should be made that the colostomy is projecting from the skin, as sometimes colostomies retract completely within the first 24 hours, with the danger that the peritoneal cavity will become contaminated with faeces. Report any of these complications immediately. It is simple for them to be corrected on the day of the operation but, if neglected, they can lead to even more serious complications.

When the first 24 hours have safely passed, the main nursing duty is to keep the skin surrounding the colostomy healthy. If the faeces are properly formed, the skin will be extremely tolerant of faecal soiling but, if the effluent from the colostomy is of diarrhoeal consistency, the skin will become reddened, inflamed and very sore, and the colostomy bag will not adhere to the skin. To prevent skin soreness, meticulous care should be taken, when changing the bag, to cut the hole in the bag to fit the stoma snugly. Before applying it to the stoma, the surrounding skin should be washed with warm soapy water and dried thoroughly. Tinc. Benz. Co. (compound tincture of benzoin, or Friar's balsam)should then be applied to produce a 'tacky' surface to which the bag will adhere. The daily change of plaster required may make the skin sore anyway, and the modern colostomy appliance (Figure 83) has proved valuable in alleviating this. It is wise to check with the patient that the adhesive surface of the bag does not ride up into folds, because if it does, faeces will find their way underneath it.

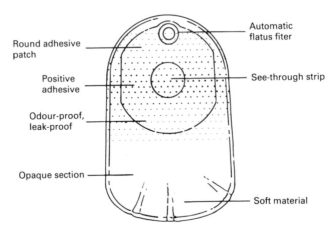

Figure 83 A modern colostomy appliance

It is easier to manage a colostomy in the left iliac fossa than one in the transverse colon. The reason is that a transverse colostomy discharges semi-fluid faeces continuously because there is little water-absorbing mucosa close to it. A pelvic colostomy, on the other hand, evacuates one or more formed stools per day because there is much more water-absorbing mucosa proximally. A transverse colostomy is therefore not suitable as a permanent arrangement.

The consistency of the stools varies widely according to the diet. They rapidly liquefy if a mildly laxative diet is taken, so the patient must learn which foods have undesirable side-effects, and avoid them. If the patient has practice, the permanent colostomy can be trained to act once a day and the attached bag can be dispensed with, so all that is necessary is a light dressing supported by a belt or roll-on. Diarrhoea can be corrected by giving *codeine phosphate* tablets (30 mg three times daily) and by adding bulk-producing granules (such as *normacol* or *isogel*) to the diet.

The patient should be taught to manage his colostomy as soon as possible, especially if it is permanent. He should learn to change the bag and wash the skin, and will rapidly become expert. The patient should be given the opportunity to join the Colostomy Association before he leaves the hospital. (For excellent comprehensive text on Stoma Care see Breckman, 1981 in Further Reading on p. 169.)

Complications

Retraction is a common complication of colostomy, but the opposite (*prolapse*)may occur. Occasionally *stenosis* (over-contraction) of the colostomy occurs owing to the contraction of the subcutaneous fibrous tissue. All three conditions require surgical intervention, when the colostomy can be refashioned.

Closure of colostomy

All temporary colostomies are eventually closed. The timing of the closure is important, and is not attempted until the colon distal to the colostomy has returned to normal and is entire and free of obstruction. If there is any obstruction in the distal colon, the colostomy closure will inevitably break down and discharge faeces. Although it is a minor procedure, colostomy closure can be dangerous if the patient is not properly prepared. The colostomy wound must be healed and not infected. The lower colon should be washed out via the distal colostomy opening and via the rectum to empty it of all hard residual faeces. The concentration of organisms in the faeces is reduced by a suitable antibiotic.

After the closure, the nurse should keep a careful watch for signs and symptoms of *peritonitis* (see p. 83). A suppository should be inserted daily into the patient's rectum until the bowels are opened normally of their own accord.

Diverticular disease

A *diverticulum* is a pouch-like protrusion of mucosa through the muscle wall of the bowel at the points where the arteries pierce it (Figure 84). These may occur anywhere in the alimentary tract, but they are usually found only in the colon, and their presence there is called *diverticulosis*. It is estimated that about 25 per cent of men and women over the age of fifty have these diverticula. The reason for their occurrence is not known, but the most probable cause is an increase in pressure within the colon which pushes the mucosa through weak spots in the muscle wall. The pelvic colon is the most common site for diverticula, where it has been found that the circular muscle coat of the bowel has become greatly thickened. This muscle very readily goes into spasm, and this irregular muscle spasm is now thought to be the cause of the localized areas of high pressure within the pelvic colon which are associated with the formation of diverticula.

Diverticulosis does not normally give rise to any symptoms other than constipation. Faeces can reach the diverticula but, as these

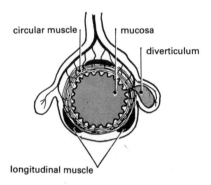

Figure 84 Cross-section of the colon in diverticular disease. The mucosa lining the colon has herniated through the circular muscle owing to abnormal pressure in the bowel

contain no muscle, they cannot contract and expel the faeces. Water is absorbed and a hard faecal concretion results, which may cause obstruction in the diverticulum. If obstruction is present, infection follows, producing the condition known as *diverticulitis*.

If a diverticulum becomes inflamed, the inflammation may spread to the pericolic tissues. The pelvic colon becomes swollen and thickened, and this may lead to a pericolic abscess, obstruction or perforation of the colon. Sometimes the inflamed colon may adhere to the bladder and cause a fistula between the pelvic colon and bladder.

Once an acute attack of diverticulitis has occurred, recurrence is common. Each attack is usually preceded by a period of constipation. In some patients the disease smoulders on and the bowel muscle, in constant spasm, becomes progressively thickened.

Symptoms

A patient with diverticulitis may come to the doctor as an acute surgical emergency with acute lower abdominal pain and fever. If perforation has occurred, the symptoms will be those of general peritonitis. Change in the bowel habit is common, and the patient may complain of increasing constipation, diarrhoea accompanied by mucus, and sometimes blood from the rectum. Occasionally, in elderly people, there may be massive bleeding of fresh blood.

Investigations

The two main investigations are sigmoidoscopy and barium enema (see Figure 81). These will demonstrate the presence of diverticula and spasm in the pelvic colon. Sometimes it is very difficult to distinguish between narrowing of the colon due to spasm and that caused by cancer of the colon. The use of the flexible sigmoidoscope has now eliminated this difficulty and is a very important advance.

Treatment

In most cases the inflammation in the colon will subside without surgical intervention, and can be treated medically. The aims are to prevent constipation, to relieve muscle spasm and to treat the infection with antibiotics. Constipation which forms hard concretions can be prevented by giving a high-residue diet, and bulk can be added to the stool by adding isogel or normacol granules. Muscle spasm is relieved by giving an antispasmodic drug such as *proban-*

thine or *colofac*. Mild inflammation is controlled by giving thalazole by mouth, but more severe attacks of inflammation will require a broad-spectrum antibiotic. Pain in diverticulitis is always relieved by pethedine. *Morphine* should never be given, because this increases muscle spasm and may cause perforation. *Pethedine*, as well as being a strong analgesic, relaxes smooth muscle and is therefore the preferred drug.

Accurate pulse and temperature charts should be maintained, as they will indicate whether the inflammation is being brought under control or if it is spreading. The administration of drugs is the nurse's responsibility, and she should also note the frequency and consistency of the stools passed. If the spasm and oedema of the colon are causing a degree of large-bowel obstruction, nasogastric suction and an intravenous drip will be necessary. If medical treatment fails, or if complications develop, surgical treatment will be necessary. For this, the pre-operative nursing care is similar to that described for previous operations.

The operation

The surgery carried out in the operating theatre will depend on what the surgeon finds when he opens the abdomen. If there is a localized peritonitis without obstruction or perforation, simple drainage will be sufficient. If there is an acute perforation, or the peritoneal cavity is contaminated with faeces, it is best to remove the diseased pelvic colon, close the rectal stump and bring out the descending colon as a terminal colostomy in the left iliac fossa. This (*Hartmann's operation*) is the ideal operation in an elderly patient. During the operation, the source of infection is removed, and the danger of performing an anastomosis on an unprepared colon is avoided. When all infection has subsided and the patient's general health is back to normal, the colon can be linked to the rectum at a second operation.

Post-operative nursing care

If a colostomy has been performed, the nursing care is as described earlier (see p. 137). The patients are usually elderly, and many also have cardiac and respiratory disabilities and are prone to pulmonary embolus (a pulmonary clot). Infection of the wound is extremely common because the operative field is infected from the outset. Particular attention needs to be paid to breathing exercises and the early mobilization of the patient. The wound must be meticulously cared for, and the drainage tubes should not be shortened or removed except under the doctor's instruction. However, drain sites should be inspected frequently and soaked dressings changed.

Chronic diverticulitis

If the disease lingers on and the symptoms are continuous or if a co-existent carcinoma cannot be excluded with certainty, the pelvic colon must be resected and the descending colon is joined to the rectum.

Pre-operative nursing care

The patient is admitted to hospital five days before the operation and a full bowel preparation is instituted with the object of providing an empty, sterile colon for the operation. Any anaemia and electrolyte imbalance must be corrected before the operation with blood and fluid transfusions.

Post-operative nursing care

The chief danger in the post-operative period is of leakage from the new anastomosis. Signs and symptoms of shock, and of an acute abdominal emergency, will alert the nurse to this event.

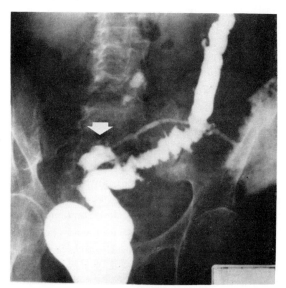

Figure 85 X-ray of post-operative rectografin enema, showing slight leakage at anastomosis at the rectosigmoid junction

Other nursing care will be as before, for major abdominal surgery.

A drain is always left *in situ* and is not removed until a *rectografin enema* (Figure 85) is given on the tenth day after the operation. This X-ray will indicate whether or not the anastomosis has healed. Always observe the drain site for faecal discharge.

In recent years, a new operation has been devised, *sigmoid myotomy*. In chronic diverticulitis, the circular muscle of the colon becomes very thickened and spastic (rigid) and, in this operation, the circular muscle is incised down as far as (but not including) the mucosa over the thickened part of the colon. The mucosa then bulges out in exactly the same way as in a *Rammstedt's operation* for pyloric stenosis of infancy (see p. 66). It is a much simpler operation than resection, and doctors await with interest the long-term results.

Ulcerative colitis

Ulcerative colitis is a disease of the mucous membrane of the colon. Its cause is unknown, and it is more common in women than in men. It is sometimes called the psychosomatic disease because the patients are usually very sensitive and introspective, but psychotherapy has no lasting effect. When the diseased colon is removed, these patients cope with an ileostomy life admirably.

The disease always starts in the rectum, where the mucous membrane is destroyed and large shallow areas of ulceration are formed (Figure 86). The disease normally runs a fluctuating course – an active phase lasting for weeks or months is followed by a quiescent period lasting for a longer or shorter time. When the disease is quiescent, an attempt is made to heal the ulcerated areas, but the normal mucosa is never reformed. The tiny areas of remaining normal mucosa hypertrophy and look like polypi. They are not true polypi, and are called *pseudopolypi*. If they are present for more than ten years, they may become malignant. The inflammation gradually spreads beyond the mucosa into the muscle layers of the colon, causing oedema. When this heals, fibrosis occurs and eventually the colon and rectum become narrow and rigid, like a hose-pipe. Normally, the whole colon is affected in the disease process. There are several different forms of the disease and we recognize several different clinical types

In the *mild form*, patients suffer from recurrent attacks of diarrhoea, which are never very disabling. Between attacks, they lead

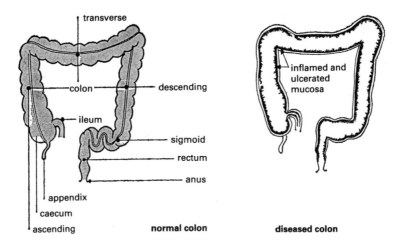

Figure 86 Extensive ulcerative colitis. The entire colon and rectum and a small portion of the terminal ileum are affected: these areas are shortened and featureless and have an inflamed, ulcerated mucosa

a perfectly normal life. Eventually the disease may burn itself out, or it may progress to a more severe form. In the *severe form*, the patient has constant diarrhoea and haemorrhage, becoming anaemic and losing weight. The *fulminating form* is the most dangerous type of ulcerative colitis. Apart from the dangers of a continuous flow of blood from the rectum, the colon may dilate rapidly and perforate. This type of colitis is often fatal.

Symptoms

Diarrhoea is the chief symptom, since the mucous membrane is destroyed to a greater or lesser degree. In addition, mucus, pus and blood are passed from the rectum. The patient may complain of weakness from the resulting anaemia and, in severe cases, weight loss, pyrexia (fever) and malaise are usual.

Investigations

There may be few physical signs on examination. Sigmoidoscopy and barium enema examination (see Figure 81) are the two diagnostic investigations necessary in every case. At sigmoidoscopy the mucous membrane is seen to be reddened, granular and ulcerated in places and, in the active stage of the disease, the lumen contains blood, mucus and pus. No preparation is needed, as this is a diagnostic sigmoidoscopy. A biopsy of the mucous membrane is always taken.

Treatment

All cases of ulcerative colitis are treated medically in the first instance. Medical treatment has three aims. Firstly, the diarrhoea must be relieved *Kaolin* and *codeine phosphate* are valuable drugs, and *isogel* and *celevac* help to retain water and diminish the fluidity of the stools. Fruit and other foods likely to produce diarrhoea are avoided. Continued diarrhoea will result in wasting, so a high-protein diet is desirable. In some cases, milk and milk products seem to aggravate the disease and it is worth eliminating these from the diet to see if this hastens recovery. Secondly, the blood loss must be corrected. Iron is given routinely but, in severe cases, blood transfusion will be necessary. Thirdly, an attempt is made to heal the inflammation in the colon and rectum. The two drugs used are *salazopyrine* (a non-specific anti-inflammatory agent given in tablet form) and *cortisone*, which is the most important drug used in the medical treatment of ulcerative colitis. Cortisone may arrest the inflammatory process altogether if given early in the disease, but it is a potentially dangerous drug as it may cause silent perforation of the colon. Furthermore, if the patient has an associated peptic ulcer, this may perforate during cortisone therapy. Therefore the nurse should constantly watch for any progressive rise in pulse rate or increasing abdominal distension. Any abnormalities must be reported at once. If cortisone is going to prove beneficial, it will soon be apparent and, if the patient's clinical state does not improve after two to three weeks' treatment, the drug should be discontinued.

Cortisone may be given in several forms. *Hydrocortisone acetate* is given by intramuscular injection or orally in tablet form as *prednisone* or *prednisolone* tablets. It can also be given as a retention enema (the *predsol retention enema*), where it acts locally on the mucosa of the rectum.

Surgical treatment

If the medical treatment fails to control the symptoms, and they are progressive, the patient will die unless surgery is carried out. This involves the excision of the entire colon and the formation of a permanent *ileostomy*. Surgery is also indicated if the disease has been present for more than ten years and the patient is in constant poor health from recurrent anaemia. In these cases, there is a risk of cancer of the colon if the disease is allowed to continue. In rare cases, emergency surgery may need to be carried out for perforation or exsanguinating haemorrhage (complete blood loss). However, these carry a high mortality. If the rectum is not involved, it may be possible to join the terminal ileum to the rectum and avoid the inconvenience of an ileostomy. If, however, the rectal stump continues to discharge pus and blood, it too must be removed. This is known as a *pan protocolectomy*.

Pre-operative nursing care

The patient should be in the best possible mental and physical condition before the operation. He may be depressed and worried, so the nurse should emphasise the positive aspects of the surgery, and reassure him that he will be able to live a much more normal life once the initial difficulties have been surmounted.

The bowel is prepared as described earlier (see p. 137). Any anaemia should be corrected by blood transfusion. If the patient has had steroids in the past year, the dose must be boosted on the day before the operation. This is very important, because it enables him to cope with the stress of operation.

Post-operative nursing care

An ileostomy is quite different from a colostomy. After resection of the terminal ileum and colon, the ileum is led out of the body as a spout ileostomy in the right iliac fossa (Figure 87). The ileostomy bag is placed in position when the patient is in the operating

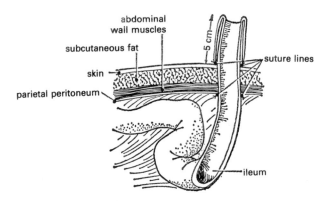

Figure 87 Structure of an ileostomy

theatre. The discharge is liquid, and contains the digestive enzymes of the small intestine. When the patient comes back from the operating theatre, the volume of the effluent from the ileostomy should be measured and recorded on the fluid balance chart. Blood pressure readings should be taken every hour. If the blood pressure is not maintained, the dosage of steroids may have to be increased. The wound is often slow to heal, particularly if the patient is on large doses of steroids. Abdominal and perineal wounds should be carefully watched, and the dressings should be changed as frequently as necessary.

The enzymes which are discharged from the ileostomy will severely *excoriate* (make sore) the skin if they come into contact with it. This excoriation is extremely difficult to heal, and the ileostomy should be looked after carefully to ensure that no excoriation takes place. Any redness or excoriation round the ileostomy stoma should be reported at once. The modern ileostomy bag makes nursing care easier. There are many varieties available, but in all of them the skin around the ileostomy is covered with adhesive plaster to which the bag is attached (Figure 88). Modern adhesives are so efficient that ileostomy fluid cannot seep between it and the skin. An ileostomy should project about two and a half centimetres from the skin in the form of a spout so that the discharge goes directly into the bag. When the bag is full, it may be emptied by a tap at the lower end without needing to remove the complete appliance. A well-fitted bag should be changed only at weekly intervals. However, when it is first fitted, the bag may slip, and the nurse should watch out for this.

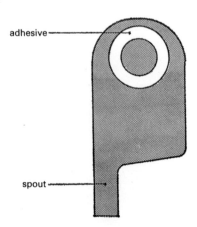

Figure 88 An ileostomy bag. The neck of the bag is applied to the skin around the ileostomy, which itself protrudes through the neck into the bag

The patient will be encouraged to know that bathing will not interfere with the ileostomy equipment, which will remain adherent provided the water is not too hot. Bathing will also assist the healing of the perineum.

The patient will be encouraged to look after his own ileostomy as soon as possible so that he will be ready to make the difficult transition from hospital to home. An ileostomy is more difficult to regulate than a colostomy. The consistency of the effluent is at first very fluid and indeed large volumes of small-bowel fluid may be lost during the first ten days. After that, the consistency should be maintained by dieting, aiming at a full, mixed diet. Patients soon learn which foods upset them.

Rehabilitation of these patients can start in hospital. They should read the booklet 'The Care of Your Ileostomy', and should be encouraged to join the Ileostomy Society of Great Britain and Ireland. (Please refer to Breekman, 1981 for detailed care.)

Carcinoma of the colon

Carinoma of the colon is a common condition. It is more common in men than in women and, although it can occur at any age, it is most common in the elderly. Of all cancers that occur in the large bowel, about half are found in the rectum; the next most common site is the pelvic colon (Figure 89). Carcinoma of the caecum and ascending colon account for most of the remainder.

A carcinoma of the colon may arise from apparently normal bowel epithelium or in a benign polyp (over two-thirds of patients with a carcinoma of the colon or rectum have an associated benign

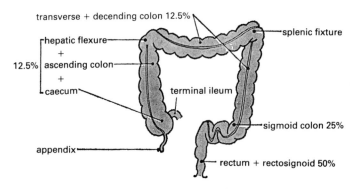

Figure 89 The distribution of carcinomas in the colon

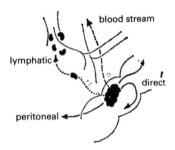

Figure 90 The spread of carcinoma of the colon

polyp nearby). People with long-standing ulcerative colitis have an increased liability to carcinoma. In rare cases, the disease may be inherited (*familial* or *hereditary polyposis of the colon*) and, of these sufferers, nearly half will die.

What does a cancer of the colon look like? There are several types of carcinoma of the colon which can be recognized with the naked eye. The *polypoidal* type looks like a cauliflower and projects into the lumen of the bowel. This type is seen commonly in the caecum, and also in the rectum. The *malignant ulcer* is more serious, and usually grows around the complete circumference of the bowel. This type will eventually cause obstruction. The *malignant stricture* (sometimes called a 'ring carcinoma', because it looks as if a string has been drawn tightly around the bowel) is usually a small cancer but it can cause obstruction early.

Like a carcinoma elsewhere in the body, cancer of the colon first spreads by local invasion. When the growth reaches the surface of the bowel, it can spread quickly into the surrounding fat and adjacent organs (Figure 90). Another common method of spread is via the blood stream. Death from cancer of the bowel is nearly always due to secondary cancers develping in the liver via the portal venous system.

Carcinoma of the caecum and ascending colon

Patients with carcinoma of the caecum or the ascending colon often suffer from anaemia. A carcinoma in this region is usually large and polypoidal, constantly exuding small quantities of blood. This is so intimately mixed with the faeces that it is not noticed by the patient. Anaemia will cause weakness, lassitude and pallor, and the patient may notice the presence of a lump. Obstruction is seldom noticed at first, because the right side of the colon is very distensible and the contents are fluid.

Carcinoma of the transverse colon

Patients suffering from this disorder most commonly come to the doctor with obstruction. However, before the obstructive symptoms develop, there is usually a history of alteration in the bowel habit.

Carcinoma of the descending and pelvic colon

This is the most common site for a carcinoma of the colon. Any recent disturbance in the bowel habit generally indicates that the patient is harbouring a carcinoma of the colon, until proved otherwise. Generally, the nearer the growth is to the rectum, the more frequent will this symptom be. Rectal bleeding is common, and complete obstruction may occur. This is because a lump of hard faeces has become impacted in the growth, which has already narrowed the lumen. In complete large-bowel obstruction, there may be little or no pain, the only symptoms being absolute constipation and increasing abdominal distension. The patient may feel well and eat normally. This is in contrast to acute small-bowel obstruction.

Carcinoma of the rectum

This is the most common site of cancer in the whole of the large bowel, the malignant ulcer being the usual variety. There is no pain until the cancer reaches the anal canal, where there is a rich supply of nerves. Nearly 70 per cent of all rectal cancers may be felt by a digital examination. Spurious diarrhoea, rectal bleeding and tenesmus are the common symptoms.

Investigations

Every case is investigated as described earlier (see p. 130). Digital examination, sigmoidoscopy and biopsy are especially important investigations in carcinoma of the rectum. A barium enema is vital in cancers high in the colon, but is of no value in carcinoma of the rectum.

Treatment

Very careful preparation of the patient is needed before the operation, if this is to be successful. The procedure for preparation of the bowel follows closely that set out on page 137. If the patient is suffering from carcinoma of the rectum, he should be aware of the possibility that a colostomy might need to be carried out, and he should understand all about it and be suitably prepared.

The treatment aims to remove the growth and all its extensions. As in all cancer surgery, as much as possible of the lymphatic field draining the tumour is removed *en bloc* with the tumour. It is generally agreed that beyond five centimetres of normal colon on either side of the growth will be free of tumour cells.

In the absence of complications, a one-stage operation can be carried out. For growths in the caecum and ascending colon, a right *hemicolectomy* is carried out. In this operation, the last fifteen to twenty centimetres of the terminal ileum, the caecum, the ascending colon, the hepatic flexure and the proximal half of the transverse colon are resected. It is necessary to remove this amount of colon in order to clear the lymphatic field. Then, an end-to-end anastomosis is carried out between the ileum and the distal half of the transverse colon.

For carcinoma of the rectum, additional pre-operative preparation needs to be carried out. In addition to the routine bowel preparation, a catheter should always be passed before the operation. This is because, after any operation deep in the pelvis, the patient will experience difficulty in micturition for the first five days.

For growths of the upper rectum, it is usually possible to completely remove the growth and to anastomose the descending colon to the lower rectum. This is known as an *anterior resection* of the rectum. For growths in the lower rectum, it is impossible to preserve the anal mechanism. For any tumour within ten centi-

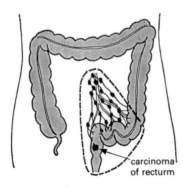

carcinoma of recturm

Figure 91 Abdomino-perineal resection for carcinoma of the rectum. The lower part of the rectum, and canal and lymph nodes are removed *en bloc*

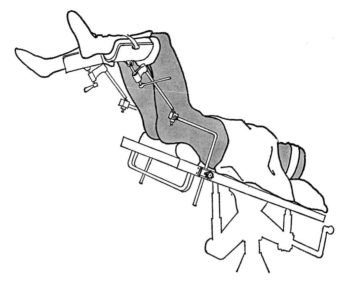

Figure 92 The position of the patient for abdomino–perineal resection of the rectum

metres of the anus, an anastomosis is impossible and an *abdomino-perineal resection* of the rectum must be carried out, with a permanent left-iliac colostomy established (Figures 91 and 92). This operation is carried out by two surgeons working together. One surgeon operates from the abdomen, the other from the perineum. The whole rectum and anal canal are removed, together with the associated lymph drainage area.

Post-operative nursing care

The patient is returned to the ward with a nasogastric tube, an intravenous drip and an abdominal drain in position. A broad-spectrum antibiotic will be given for at least five days, an accurate fluid balance chart should be maintained, and the pulse and temperature should be accurately recorded. These give an early warning of any complications. The patient may have 30 ml of water hourly, but no solid food should be given until the bowels are opened normally. A normal bowel action means that the anastomosis has healed.

Breakdown of the anastomosis is a dangerous complication which can occur at any time up to ten days after the operation. It is for this reason that a drainage tube is always left in situ, and this should not be removed or shortened without the surgeon's instructions. If there are no complications, the amount of drainage decreases daily.

If pus begins to drain, this may mean that a leak has occurred at the anastomosis, so it should be reported immediately. However, a slight leak is not serious – it will drain to the surface and always closes in a short while. The wound dressing should not be disturbed unless the wound is painful, tender or discharging. If a catheter is in position, it should be removed on the morning of the fifth day. If retention occurs, then it should be replaced for a further period.

Post-operative pain, especially during the first 48 hours, may be relieved by strong analgesics such as pethedine or omnopon, given by intramuscular injection. From the third day onwards, a suppository should be inserted into the rectum daily to encourage restoration of normal bowel function.

Following an abdomino-perineal resection of the rectum, it will be necessary to care for the colostomy as well as the abdominal wound. This is discussed in detail on page 137 and in *Stoma Care* (Breckman, 1981). The care of the perineal wound is very important. Primary closure of the perineal skin is usually carried out. The large cavity beneath this wound quickly fills up with blood and serum, so it is always drained with a corrugated rubber tube or by suction drainage. However, the drainage may become obstructed by clots and, if these are not removed, they will become infected and seriously delay healing. The nurse may be asked to irrigate the perineal wound once or twice daily to prevent accumulation of clots and debris. The solution used will depend upon the individual patient and should be checked either with the ward sister or the surgeon as appropriate. It will help to take the strain off the perineal skin if the patient lies on his side. It is vital to be scrupulous in the care of the perineum. It is a moist area which is always slow to heal and, if it becomes badly infected, it may delay the patient's departure from hospital by many weeks. During the first ten days after the operation, the patient may be very depressed and will need reassurance that, in time, he can return to leading a normal life. A visitor from the Colostomy Association may well encourage him, both now and before the operation takes place. As soon as possible, the patient should learn to manage his own colostomy, and the visitor from the Colostomy Welfare Group can often help in advising the patient about the most suitable type of colostomy apparatus. In many hospitals now there is also a stoma care nurse, who will provide specific advice and expertise to these patients. All patients will need to convalesce, and arrangements with a convalescence hospital should be made in good time.

There are two important complications which may occur in carcinoma of the large bowel. These are *obstruction* and *perforation*.

Obstruction

If the patient is acutely obstructed and enemata fail to relieve the obstruction, an emergency *laparotomy* (surgical opening of the abdomen) is carried out. Resection and anastomosis is very hazardous in the presence of obstruction, so a colostomy proximal to the obstructing growth is fashioned. This colostomy is opened in the operating theatre, thereby relieving the obstruction. The patient's general condition may now be improved and the colon prepared in the usual way. At a second operation, the carcinoma is removed, and a third operation will be necessary to close the colostomy. These will take anything up to three months, and elderly patients may well develop respiratory and cardiac complications during this time. A one-stage operation is preferable for these people.

Perforation

Fortunately this is rare. The signs and symptoms are those of a generalized peritonitis, and emergency laparotomy, drainage and colostomy are required.

Patients with advanced cancer which cannot be removed can still be helped, and their pain, suffering and obstruction may be relieved. An anastomosis between the part of the bowel above and that below the tumour will relieve the obstruction. In cases of carcinoma of the rectum, even if the liver is full of secondary deposits, it is preferable to remove the rectum, if this is possible. To leave the growth *in situ* results in considerable distress from *tenesmus* and constant discharge of blood and pus.

Ten

The anal canal

The anal canal is just under four centimetres long, and is surrounded by very important muscles called *sphincters* (Figure 93). Like the colon, the wall of the anal canal has longitudinal and circular muscle layers but, in the anal canal, the layer of circular muscle becomes thickened to form the *internal sphincter*. The *external sphincter* is a complex arrangement formed partly by a continuation of the longitudinal muscle of the colon and partly by the *levator ani* muscles. These muscles form the muscular part of the pelvic floor and are the most powerful muscles controlling the pelvic outlet. If they are not functioning properly, collapse of the floor (*prolapse*) will result.

The anal canal has an elaborate muscosal lining. The upper half of the canal is lined by *columnar epithelium*, the lower half by *stratified squamous epithelium* (Figure 94). The two halves of the anal canal have different blood supplied (Figure 95), different lymphatic drainage and different nerve supplies.

In the upper half of the anal canal, venous blood drains upwards to the *superior haemorrhoidal vessels* of the rectum (Figure 96) and from there to the portal system of veins. The lymph vessels also drain upwards. The nerve supply is via the autonomic nervous

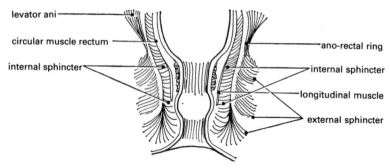

Figure 93 The muscles of the anal canal

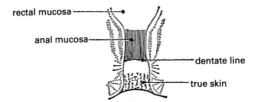

Figure 94 The lining of the anal canal

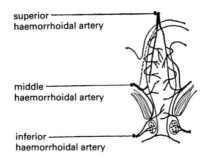

Figure 95 The blood supply of anal canal

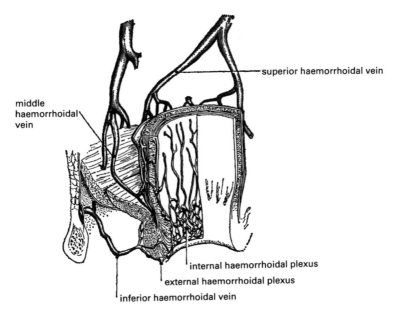

Figure 96 The venous drainage of the rectum

system alone, so the lining of the lining of the upper anal canal is relatively insensitive.

In the lower half of the canal, venous blood drains downwards to the *inferior haemorrhoidal vein*. Lymph vessels drain to glands in the groin. The nerve supply is via the somatic nerves, so the lower anal canal is very sensitive and any lesion is extremely painful.

The space between the lining mucosa and the internal sphincter muscle in the upper half of the anal canal is called the *submucous space*. This is where internal haemorrhoids occur. External haemorrhoids occur beneath the skin of the lower half of the anal canal. At the junction of the upper and lower parts of the anal canal the mucous membrane is pitted or *serrated*. These serrations are *anal crypts*, into which *anal glands* open. If these glands become infected, they may give rise to fistulae and fissures.

Any disease of the lower half of the anal canal will cause pain, because the muscosa is so sensitive. A swelling may be present which could be an internal haemorrhoid which has prolapsed, a *perianal haematoma* resulting from thrombosis in an external haemorrhoid, an abscess, or a skin tag (which results from shrivelling of an external haemorrhoid). Irritation is a common symptom and results from soiling with faeces or the passage of mucus. Bleeding at the time of defaecation occurs if a damaged area is grazed by the passage of a stool. This occurs commonly in haemorrhoids.

Examination of the anal canal is a straightforward procedure. Most lesions are visible or easily felt on digital examination with the gloved finger. The *proctoscope* is a simple tube, about five centimetres long, which can be inserted into the anal canal to inspect the mucosa for the presence of haemorrhoids and other lesions. No special investigations are necessary.

There are several common disorders of the anal canal. Although these are rarely serious, they can be both painful and inconvenient.

Haemorrhoids

The term haemorrhoid is often ascribed by the layman to any lump which appears at the anal orifice. In fact, true internal haemorrhoids (*piles*) are dilated veins occurring in the submucous space in the anal canal and they occupy definite sites (Figure 97). One site is in the left lateral position, the other two occupy the right anterior and posterior sites. They correspond to the terminations of the *superior haemorrhoidal vessels*.

internal   external

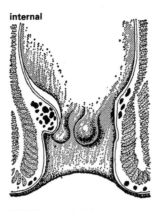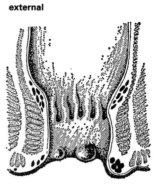

Figure 97 Haemorrhoids

The cause of haemorrhoids is unknown. They can arise in patients in their teens, but they are more common in middle age. At every act of defaecation there is some prolapse of the mucosa but, if the bowels are constipated, there will be excessive congestion of the superior haemorrhoidal veins at each bowel movement. This can easily lead to the formation of dilatations or varicosities in the veins.

Haemorrhoids are classified into three groups. In *first degree* haemorrhoids, bleeding is the only symptom because the mucosa covering the early haemorrhoid is easily injured by the passage of a stool. In *second degree* haemorrhoids, the dilated part of the vein prolapses every time defaecation occurs, but returns to the anal canal spontaneously after defaecation. In *third degree* haemorrhoids the dilated veins prolapse not only on defaecation, but every time pressure inside the abdomen is raised, such as when lifting heavy objects or in late pregnancy. Because the dilated vein does not return to its position spontaneously, it has to be replaced manually. Patients with third degree haemorrhoids are never really free from discomfort.

The main symptom of uncomplicated haemorrhoids is bleeding. The blood is bright red in colour and occurs only when stools are passed. If the bleeding recurs, it may give rise to severe anaemia. When the haemorrhoids prolapse, patients usually complain of a lump at the edge of the anus, accompanied by a dull, aching sensation. The damage mucosa can secrete mucus, which seeps on to the skin and irritates the anus.

As with any other lesion in the gastro-intestinal tract, complications can occur. *Strangulation* of a haemorrhoid is the most important complication. First of all, the haemorrhoid prolapses. If the internal sphincter goes into spasm, it will partially cut off its blood supply. Thromboses (clots) will then appear in the haemorrhoidal veins, and the surrounding tissues will become inflamed. This sequence of events leads to an extremely tender and painful swelling at the edge of the anus, as the lower half of the anal canal is richly supplied with somatic nerves. If infection now takes place, it can (in theory) spread to the liver via the portal vein, but this is extremely rare.

Treatment

First and second degree haemorrhoids are normally treated by the injection of a *sclerosant* solution during an out-patient procedure called *sclerotherapy*, in which the veins are hardened up. The solution usually used is 5 per cent phenol in almond oil. A proctoscope is inserted into the anal canal and the haemorrhoids identified. Then, about 3 ml of the sclerosant solution are injected into the submucous space at the topmost part of each pile. A special type of syringe with a long needle is used. The nurse should prepare the syringes and fill them with the correct solution. The name of the solution should be carefully checked before filling the syringes, and the label of the bottle should be shown to the doctor. The patient should understand the procedure and be reassured that it is painless because the injection is placed into the insensitive submucosa above the anal canal. If the injection is placed too low, severe pain and discomfort will occur. Sometimes patients feel weak and faint after the injections, so they should be kept under observation for a few minutes.

The solution from the syringe is injected into the submucous space in which the haemorrhoidal vessels lie. First of all blood clotting in the vein (*venous thrombosis*) occurs, followed by the formation of scar tissue (*perivenous fibrosis*). These changes prevent prolapse of the mucosa and cut down the amount of blood in the haemorrhoid, so the bleeding ceases. The injections may relieve the symptoms for many years, especially if the patient's bowel habits are normal.

If the patients do not respond to sclerotherapy, the haemorrhoids may be excised in the operation known as *haemorrhoidectomy*. Third degree haemorrhoids are usually treated in this way. The surgeon cuts the haemorrhoid and its overlying mucosa away from the internal sphincter to a point above the junction of the skin and the mucous membrane. At this point the base of the haemorrhoid is transfixed with strong non-absorbable suture material and tied off, it is then cut off below the ligature.

The three types of haemorrhoid are dealt with in exactly the same way, leaving a little column of mucosa between each area cut away. This is very important if narrowing of the anal canal is to be avoided.

Pre-operative nursing care

The aim of the nurse should be to get the anus and surrounding skin as clean as possible. First, the lower bowel should be emptied. Although the modern disposable enema is more convenient, the older soap-and-water enema is far more effective in this case. Twenty-four hours before the operation, the enema is administered, but it should be preceded by an aperient the previous evening. On the night before the operation, the patient's perianal skin and suprapubic area may need to be shaved. This depends upon the procedures in particular hospitals. The nurse will quickly become aware of these the longer she works in the area.

Post-operative nursing care

Following haemorrhoidectomy, pain can be severe. The drug omnopon in suitable doses will usually be necessary once or twice in the first 24 hours after the operation. Careful observation should be made for any sign of haemorrhage. If the bleeding is severe, a ligature may well have slipped from one of the haemorrhoid pedicles, and this should be reported at once. At one time a rubber tube was left in situ in the anal canal, but this was so uncomfortable for the patient that it is now rarely used. Good nursing and careful observation of the anal region are used instead. Mild oozing can be treated by pressure packing, but severe haemorrhage will have to be controlled in the theatre.

As soon as he feels well enough, the patient can have a normal diet, as there is no advantage in not using the bowels for five days. This only results in the eventual very painful passage of rock-hard stools. There are several oral aperients that can be regularly administered from the first day post-operatively so as to facilitate the passing of a soft stool as early as the second day post-operatively. This is essential to prevent an otherwise extremely painful experience later on, if the patient is allowed to become constipated. Hot baths should be encouraged by the nurse. These would prevent the necessity for keeping dressings on the wound, particularly if baths are taken two or three times a day. However, as always, individual patient differences should be appreciated. The nursing care should, as always, be discussed with the patient and not dictated to him.

From the fifth day onwards, digital dilatation of the anal canal is carried out by the doctor to ensure that the anal canal does not become narrowed. The patient is normally discharged from hospital on the tenth post-operative day.

Strangulated haemorrhoids

In the past, strangulated haemorrhoids were treated by complete bed rest, applications of lead and opium compresses, and analgesic drugs to relieve the pain. The inflammation and swelling usually took several weeks to subside, and it was difficult to reduce the associated prolapse because of spasm of the internal sphincter muscles. More recently, strangulated haemorrhoids have been successfully treated by dilatation of the internal sphincter under general anaesthetic. Prolapse and oedema subside within a few days. Emergency haemorrhoidectomy has also been proved to be safe, and this is probably the best treatment.

Fissure-in-ano

Of all the conditions in the anal canal, *fissure-in-ano* is the most painful. A fissure is a longitudinal ulcer in the lower half of the anal canal (Figure 98). The most common cause of this is injury to the mucosa by the passage of hard stool, which splits the lining. The

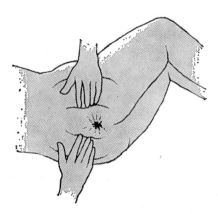

Figure 98 Fissure-in-ano

other cause is infection in an anal gland beneath the mucosa. Pus forms, and may track down beneath the skin. The overlying mucosa sloughs off, forming a fissure. As the floor of the fissure is the internal sphincter muscle, pain and muscle spasm will result. The pain is made worse by the passage of a stool, which distends the anal canal, and the acute pain may last for several hours afterwards. The patient therefore dreads defaecation, and constipation results. More and more water is absorbed by the rectal mucosa from the retained faeces and, when the bowels are eventually opened, the stools are rock hard. This will reactivate the fissure and result in a vicious circle of pain. When these patients are examined, marked spasm and tightness of the anal canal are found, which may be so severe that examination is impossible without a general anaesthetic. Muscle spasm is the factor which prevents healing of fissures and, if the spasm is overcome, healing will take place. In mild cases, a local analgesic ointment (such as *lignocaine gel*) will relieve pain if applied into the anal canal. A laxative taken by mouth will keep the stools soft and prevent further damage from hard faeces. A tube or anal dilator can be passed daily by the patient. These measures may allow complete healing to occur but, if they fail, an operation may be necessary in which the internal sphincter is partially divided. This prevents spasm and will allow healing to occur.

The post-operative nursing care is similar to that after haemorrhoidectomy (see p. 161). Healing may take several weeks, but the pain is cured immediately.

Infection in the anal canal

Anal wounds often heal completely without infection, in spite of the passage of faeces which are teeming with microorganisms. However, inflammation in the tissues around the anal canal is quite common. This is due to the anal glands, which lie beneath the mucous membrane and open into the anal canal at the junction of the upper and lower halves. If the opening of these glands becomes blocked or traumatized (damaged), they may become infected and abscesses will occur.

If the infection spreads downwards beneath the skin, a *perianal abscess* will result. If it spreads outwards through the sphincters, it will reach the fat of the *ischio-rectal space* alongside the rectum, and an *ischio-rectal abscess* will occur. The symptoms and signs will depend upon the site of the abscess, but will, of course, be most painful lower down.

Treatment

An abscess, wherever it occurs, must be incised and free drainage of the pus established.

Pre-operative nurse care

Most cases are admitted for emergency operation. No special preparation is needed, because the condition is so painful that even shaving may not be tolerated, but routine pre-operative duties should still be carried out.

Post-operative nursing care

The chief post-operative duty is to ensure that free drainage of the wound is maintained. This allows healing to occur from the bottom upwards. If the skin heals over too quickly, septic tracks may be left beneath it, and a fistula may result. Free drainage is maintained by irrigating the wound daily with antiseptic solutions, packing deep wounds with gauze impregnated with antiseptic solution, and keeping the skin edges apart with gauze packs. These should be changed at least once a day, and the patient is advised to have a daily bath before the packs are inserted. The patient's comfort will be increased if the bowels are opened daily.

Other anal disorders

Fistula-in-ano

A *fistula* is a track lined by granulation tissue connecting two surfaces lined with epithelium. In the anal canal, fistulae are usually the result of perianal infection. The mucous membrane of the anal canal is connected to the surface of the skin by the fistula (Figure 99) and, while fistulae elsewhere in the body tend to close, those in the anal canal tend to persist. The most likely reason for this is a chronic infection in the anal glands. The internal opening of the fistula is always at the junction between skin and mucous membrane in the anal canal. The track may pass outwards above, through or below the sphincter muscles to reach the skin. Depending on their relationship to the sphincters, fistulae are classed as *high* or *low* anal fistulae.

A fistula may be present without giving rise to much trouble

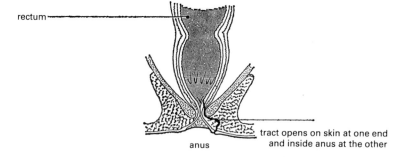

rectum

anus

tract opens on skin at one end
and inside anus at the other

Figure 99 Fistula-in-ano

apart from a slight discharge. If the track becomes blocked
however, a perianal or ischio-rectal abscess will develop.

Treatment

The principle of treatment is to excise the track leaving a wide raw
area which should heal from the bottom. The pre-operative and
post-operative nursing care is the same as that for an ischio-rectal
abscess (see p. 164). It is especially important that the skin edges
should be kept apart by dressings in the correct positions. Daily or
twice-daily baths help greatly to keep the area clean. The skin must
not be allowed to heal over before the underlying cavity has filled
up with granulation tissue. Patients can have a normal diet, and
should be encouraged to have their bowels opened daily.

In the more complicated fistulae, the surgeon may not be able
to excise the track at one operation, especially if the track traverses
the sphincter muscles. In these cases, in order to prevent permanent damage to the sphincters, the track is laid open and excised
little by little at weekly or fortnightly intervals. These are called
fistula review operations.

Rectal prolapse

When all the coats of the wall lining the rectum collapse outside
the anal canal, a condition called *rectal prolapse* occurs. It is most
commonly found in the very young and the very old. In infants,
spontaneous cure is usual, but the most frequent sufferers are
elderly women and patients in mental hospitals. The cause is not
properly understood, but certain conditions seem more likely to
result in a rectal prolapse. Chronic constipation, injury to the

perineal muscles during childbirth and weakness of the supporting ligaments in the pelvis with advancing age are the more important ones.

Complete rectal prolapse is a very distressing condition. Patients are unable to leave the house and have to wear a pad permanently, as they are usually incontinent.

Many operations have been devised to cure this condition, but the recurrence rate is extremely high. It is hoped that, with increasing understanding of the function of the pelvic muscles, a more satisfactory form of treatment will not be long delayed.

Pilonidal sinus

A pilonidal sinus is a nest of hair lying in a blind pit lined with skin in the cleft between the buttocks. In people affected, one or more tiny pore-like openings are clearly visible on the skin, if the buttocks are separated. This condition is a common cause of infection and abscess formation (*pilonidal abscess*) in this area. Due to continued friction, hairs are driven into the sinus, where they coil up. If for any reason the openings are obstructed, stagnation and infection inevitably result.

Treatment

Wide excision of the sinus was once the preferred treatment. Sometimes the skin was closed immediately, but the recurrence rate was high. Alternatively, the raw area was allowed to heal from the bottom by granulation, but this necessitated long stays in hospital.

The modern method of treatment is to remove the hairs in the sinus by deroofing it and clearing out the impacted hair. Recurrence of the infection can be prevented if further hair is prevented from burrowing beneath the skin by shaving the area at weekly intervals.

Pruritus ani

This is an itching round the anus and is a symptom, not a disease in itself. Many factors can cause irritability of the perianal region but, when the patient scratches the area, this increases its sensitivity and marked inflammatory changes can result. It is difficult to break this vicious circle.

The investigation of this distressing condition involves a search for all the likely causes. The urine should always be tested for sugar to exclude diabetes. Scrpings should be taken from the skin to exclude a fungal infection. The stools should be examined for threadworms and other infestations. Anal soiling is a very common cause if the skin becomes sodden with excessive moisture, due to a fistula, prolapsed rectal mucosa or persistent diarrhoea. Lack of personal hygiene is also a common predisposing factor.

Treatment

Any local condition causing itching can be treated, and this may result in complete relief of symptoms. If no local or general cause is found, relief is obtained by establishing local anal hygiene and applying local analgesic lotions.

Further reading

Chapter One
Cope Z 1972 The Early diagnosis of the acute abdomen, 14th edn. Oxford University Press, Oxford.
Cotton Peter B Williams C B 1980 Practical Gastro-intestinal endoscopy. Blackwell Scientific, Oxford.
Cotton P et al 1973 A new look inside the gut: fibre-optic endoscopy. Nursing Mirror 136: 1968 22–3.
Tonkin R D, Parrish J A 1968 Lecture notes on Gastro-enterology. Blackwell, Oxford

Chapter Three
Stoker A 1973 Salivary tumours. Nursing Times 69: 302–5.

Chapter Four
Barlow D 1971 Malignant conditions of the oesophagus. Nursing Times 67: 979–81.

Chapter Five
Kemp R 1964 Understanding duodenal ulcer. Tavistock, London
Rose J F 1969 The medical treatment of gastric and duodenal ulcers. Nursing Times 65: 1038–40.

Chapter Six
Postle M 1971 Faecal peritonitis complicated by severe chest injuries – a patient care study. Nursing Times: 67 630–33.

Chapter Seven
Bouchier I A D 1970 Cancer of the Pancreas. Nursing Mirror 130: 25–7.

Chapter Eight
Bolam R F 1969 Intestinal obstruction. Nursing Times 65: 813–15.
Knight R 1972 Intestinal parasitic infections in Britain. Nursing Mirror 134: 33–4.

Kyle J 1972 Crohn's disease. Heinemann Medical, London

Picton S J 1970 The Management of fistulae by sump drainage. Nursing Times 66: 1035–8.

Chapter Nine

Breckman B (ed) 1981 Stoma care. Beaconsfield Publishers, Bucks.

Dawson A M et al 1971 A step forward in stoma care: (1) The medical problems, (2) The surgeon's point of view, (3) The work of the nurse stoma-therapist. Nursing Times 67: 477–81.

Jones F A, Goddings E W (eds) 1972 Management of Constipation. Blackwell Scientific, Oxford.

Milton-Thompson G J 1971 Constipation. Nursing Mirror 132: 30–33.

Williams C B 1973 Colonoscopy. Nursing Times: 69: 108–10.

Index